Hawaiian and Polynesian Miracle Health Secrets

by Robert B. Stone, Ph.D.
and Lola Stone

Parker Publishing Company, Inc.

West Nyack, New York

Library of Congress Cataloging in Publication Data

Stone, Robert B
  Hawaiian and Polynesian miracle health secrets.

  Includes index.
      1. Health.   2. Nutrition.   3. Folk medicine—
  Hawaii.   4. Folk medicine—Polynesia.   5. Cookery,
  Hawaiian.   6. Cookery, Polynesian.   I. Stone,
  Lola, joint author.   II. Title.   III. Title:
  Polynesian miracle health secrets.   [DNLM: 1. Medicine,
  Primitive—Hawaii.   2. Medicine, Primitive—Polynesia.
  WB50 AH3 S8h]
  RA776.5.S83   613   80-12215
  ISBN 0-13-384255-X

Printed in the United States of America

Me Kealoha Pumehana
to
Our *Keikis*

Dennis
Lynne
Paul
Alexis

A Word from the Authors

As the cost of medical care rises, the need increases for people to be themselves responsible for a strong resistance to disease and a high level of good health. It is natural to want to find out what healthy people are doing in order to learn their secrets of longevity.

Such exemplary people are the Hawaiians and the Polynesians of the South Pacific. These robust, life-loving men and women live longer and are relatively free of some of our most devastating diseases. Their health and vitality win the admiration of people all over the world.

What is it about their life style, their habits, their food, their drink and their medical practices that the rest of us can benefit from by adopting?

We have spent the past ten years living on the islands of Hawai'i, working and enjoying paradise with the local people and studying their culture and their ways. We have traveled to other islands of Polynesia like Samoa, Fiji and Tahiti, and other islands of the Pacific like Honshu, and as far as Java and Bali.

What we have learned about the natural health secrets of this fabulous part of the world can fill a book—the one you have in your hands.

We have included no herbs or plants that are not available in the mainland United States. We have included common items, fairly easily obtainable and adaptable by you whether you live in the North or South, on the coast or inland.

Here are health secrets, many unveiled for the first time, that can add years to your life. From cuts and bruises to colds and cancer, Hawaiians have natural remedies that work for them. Now they can work for you.

Fruits, greens, nuts, berries, herbs and vegetables that have special healing value are unveiled for all to use. In addition, nature has surrounded us with other avenues to better health that the Hawaiian *kahunas* (medicine men) are now willing to reveal.

A WORD FROM THE AUTHORS

The population of Hawai'i is increasing as people flock to one of the healthiest places to live on earth. On the pages ahead is your share of Hawaiian health. With this book you can make your own home a Pacific health spa for a longer and fuller life.

Robert B. Stone, Ph.D.
Lola Stone

Acknowledgments

For their valuable assistance in researching material for this book, we wish to thank the following: Edwin H. Bryan, Jr., of the Pacific Sciences Information Center of the Bishop Museum; Mrs. Katherine Bazore Gruelle for the use of some recipes from her book, *Hawaiian and Pacific Foods*; the Public Health Nursing Board of Hawai'i's State Department of Health; the Cooperative Extension Service of the University of Hawaii; Steven Taussig, Ph.D.; Mrs. Genevieve Nahulu, Kawika Bray, Karla Kral, Bob Samson, Rosita Kalsbeek, Ampi Uyehara, Imo Tiapula, Henry Yamamoto, and many others who have shared their cultural and family secrets with us.

Contents

5. Life-Giving Island Fruits and Nuts Available Everywhere **93**

The "Fruit of Paradise" (96)
The Tenderizer Fruit (99)
The Fruit Without a Tree (100)
Ananas Are Not Bananas (102)
A Fruit for the Starving (104)
Your Tropical Fruit Bowl (105)
Hawai'i's Health Nuts (107)
The Palm Tree's Contribution to Health (108)
A Special Oil for the Body (109)
Other Hawaiian and Polynesian Nuts Your Body Can
    Enjoy (109)

6. Other Foods Hawaiians and Polynesians Eat to Stay Young **113**

The Hawaiian and Polynesian "Staff of Life" (116)
Valuable Vegetables from the Sea (118)
How to Obtain Seaweed Without Getting Your Feet Wet
    (120)
The Bean That Does a Steak's Job (122)
A High Protein Seasoning (124)
A High Protein Sauce (125)
The Meaning of Green to Hawaiian and Polynesian
    Peoples (127)
Sprouting Better Health (128)
An Antacid from Japan (129)

7. Polynesian Health Practices That Work Anywhere **131**

Vital Energy and Its Control by Breath (134)
The Real Meaning Behind Fijian Fire Walking (136)
How to Freshen the Air You Breathe (137)
Fresh Drinking Water—Its Importance to Your Health
    (140)
Other Drinks—And What to Avoid (141)
The Frosty Delight That Hawaiians Enjoy (142)

1

You Can Enjoy the Longer Life of Hawaiians and Polynesians

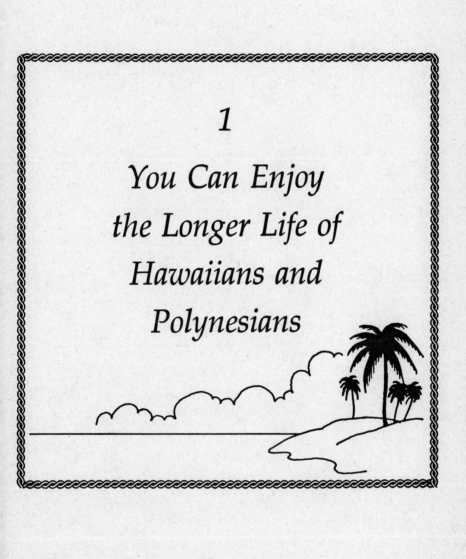

The lilting music of *ukuleles,* the swaying hips of dancing maidens, and voices singing of the beauty of the islands are unmistakable images of Hawai'i.

Hawaiians, as well as other Polynesians, may have a good reason to sing, dance and celebrate: They live longer than anyone else in the world.

According to a recent report in the *Hawaii Medical Journal,* "A baby girl born here in 1975 and living here under unchanging 1975 mortality conditions would have an expected life of almost 78 years, while a baby boy would live 74 years. These values are probably the highest in the United States and are among the highest in the world." The infant mortality rate in the U.S. was 15.2 per 1000 in 1977. In Hawai'i it was 10.6—30 percent less.

Unlike the Hunzas of Kashmir, who have gained a reputation for longevity by dint of a few people who have lived to be 125 and even older, the Hawaiians produce few such centenarians today, but the life expectancy is high because everyone is at a higher level of good health.

At the end of the last century, a royal high chief named Kalanihupule, the oldest member of the Kalani family, is said to have been 180 years old when he died. Some years before, he had reportedly given away a big slice of the windward side of the island of O'ahu to a missionary family in exchange for a pair of binoculars. You may think that he must have been senile to do that, but don't bet on it. Hawaiian people have easygoing ways. They find it easy to give, easy to love, easy to have fun. And there is evidence that this characteristic may have something to do with their longer life span.

We have lived in Hawai'i for ten years. We consider ourselves to be Hawaiians just as we once considered ourselves as New Yorkers. We do not have any Hawaiian blood in our veins but neither do 83 percent of all the people who live in Hawai'i today.

The statistics pointing to the longest living people in the world are made up of people from New York, Illinois, Tennessee, California and the rest of the United States, as well as Japan, China, the Philippines and other countries.

So it is not Hawaiian blood flowing in human veins that brings a longer life, but rather the Hawaiian life style. This way of life adds years to the lives of people from any culture, any country and any race.

What are the essential aspects of the Hawaiian way of life that produce health, vitality and longevity?

What foods, what medicines, what activities contribute to Hawaiian well-being?

This book reveals the answers to these questions, and the answers make these higher levels of well-being available to you wherever you live.

THE NATURE OF HAWAIIAN HEALTH SECRETS

The *Canadian Medical Association Journal,* as early as 1938, pointed out that potassium produced a decline in blood pressure, while sodium produced an increase in blood pressure.

It has taken 50 years for medical researchers to find that the potassium in bananas lowers the blood pressure by flushing excess salt—sodium—out of the body.

Hawaiians do not say, "A banana a day keeps the doctor away," but Hawaiians love their bananas, and bananas are certainly one of the reasons why Hawai'i's death rate in 1977 was 4.9 per 1000 residents, almost half the national rate (9.1).

Millions of Americans are dying needlessly of cardiovascular problems.

Now the secret is out about bananas. Hopefully, you will look at bananas differently from now on when you see them in the supermarket.

Scores and scores of other Hawaiian and Polynesian health secrets are just as accessible to you as bananas. (Incidentally, we'll say more about the other health benefits of bananas in Chapter 5.)

In fact, bananas are not the only answer to the threat of high blood pressure. Also high in potassium are watermelon, cantaloupe and many vegetables which have been only lightly cooked. They contain the same potassium, ready to flush excess salt from the body and keep blood pressure at healthier levels.

As we bring the health secrets of the Hawaiian people to you, you will begin to see a pattern. At first you will put a big exclamation point opposite bananas on your shopping list. Then you will add another item to your shopping list, or two, or three. But one day you will say, "Ah, hah!" And that will be the day you really grasp the Hawaiian life style.

From that day on, you will be living each day in a more Hawaiian way. You will be living each day happier and healthier. And you will have more days to live.

WELLNESS VERSUS SICKNESS

In March 1979, thousands gathered in Honolulu for a wellness celebration. Called *Pono Maka'i*, it was based on a definition of wellness adopted a few months earlier by the Hawaiian Statewide Health Coordinating Council:

> The wellness way of living is a lifestyle you design to achieve your best potential for well-being, encompassing nutrition, physical vitality, and emotional stability. It involves your whole being—physical, mental, emotional, spiritual— and how you relate to your environment.

Present at the celebration were both lay and professional people, sharing their expertise in the personal integration of wellness concepts and skills. It was quite different from the typical medical meeting. Booths and workshops were not devoted to new drugs, new pain relievers or new antacids. These booths and workshops featured nutrition, exercise, relaxation, recreation, stress management, creativity, personal safety and hygiene.

Hawaiians are less oriented to sickness and its cure than they are to wellness and its enjoyment. They prefer a treat to a treatment.

You do not have to be "transplanted" to Hawai'i to feel the same way.

Bill Y. ran a small print shop in a suburb of Chicago. Business got better and better. And Bill got worse and worse. There was more machinery to buy in order to keep up with the growing volume, more bills to pay and more accounts to collect. His wife kept telling him to slow down. His doctor kept telling him to slow down. Finally, his body, which had also been telling him to slow down, "put its foot down." Bill had a mild heart attack.

He and his wife decided to sell their home and business and move to Hawai'i, where their son was stationed in the military. There Bill did some consulting work in the mornings but spent the rest of the day playing his favorite game of lawn bowling (see Chapter 10) and swimming and sunning at the beach.

Today he looks ten years younger, is at the peak of good health, and is enjoying life like never before.

What caused the change in Bill? The sunning? The bowling? The swimming? Maybe. But they were merely the means to an end.

The means to the same end are available everywhere. What you will learn from the nature of Hawaiian and Polynesian health secrets are not the monopoly of those islands in the Pacific. They can be applied successfully on your "island"—the home in which you reside, the community in which you work, and the environment in which you live.

All it really takes is an awareness of wellness, in place of a fear of sickness, and a knowledge of the sources of "not wellness."

That is what this book is all about.

The nation's three worst killers are heart disease, cancer and stroke. In Hawai'i they make less headway:

Deaths per 100,000 in 1977

	Heart Disease	Cancer	Stroke
United States	336	171	80
Hawai'i	148	125	40

Hawaiians and Polynesians can teach you a thing or two about wellness.

YOUR GROWING RESPONSIBILITY
FOR YOUR OWN HEALTH

In Hawai'i there is a Planning Task Force for wellness.

One of the largest hospitals in Hawai'i conducts a Healthing Clinic to keep healthy people healthy.

The Hawai'i Medical Service Association, one of the leading medical insurance plans, conducts ongoing educational programs in wellness.

This is not happening in Hawai'i alone. Throughout the United States there are growing numbers of conferences for wellness-oriented professionals; cruises and weekend retreats for health-conscious people; and holistic health centers where the whole person—body, mind and spirit—receives integration and reinforcement.

We are all in the same boat. We are faced with the spiraling costs of medical care. Many of us have lost personal contact with our physicians because of their busy schedules, specialized tests and technicians. We are repeatedly confronted with the fact that we are risking possibly fatal diseases by behaviors and life styles that are largely under our own personal control.

We are going to have to row and steer that boat. As hospitals become full, as costs continue to rise, as national resources devoted to health become more thinly spread, as the delivery of health care to growing numbers of sick people becomes increasingly difficult, we are going to have to take charge of ourselves—as Hawaiians and Polynesians have been doing for centuries.

We are going to have to know what makes us sick and what keeps us healthy. And what better place to learn than where people stay the healthiest and live the longest!

It has taken us ten years to learn. We are ready to teach you in ten hours.

THE JOY OF PRACTICING ISLAND HEALTH SECRETS

What you learn will be easy to take.

Do you think for one minute that Hawaiians are living a life of diet, sacrifice and chastity?

The Hawaiian life is a life of pleasure and joy.

Hawaiian wellness includes plenty of good food, plenty of good drink, plenty of fun both indoors and outdoors.

If anything, adopting Hawaiian and Polynesian health secrets will mean for you a shift from boredom, drudgery, tension and worry, to getting more done in less time with greater energy, enthusiasm and fun.

Charlotte L. decided that if she could be a good typist in New York, she could be a good typist in Hawai'i. And maybe the move would help her sinus condition and repeated cold and flu attacks. When she started to look for work, she discovered that jobs in Hawai'i are not that easy to find and usually pay less than equivalent skills in large mainland cities.

While Charlotte was job hunting, week after week, she was also finding a new way to face life. She was meeting Hawaiian people, eating the Hawaiian way and adopting a Hawaiian life style. In six months her money ran out and she had to go back to New York. She got her old job back. But now things were different. She kept her Hawaiian ways and her sinus, colds and flus did not return. She enjoyed a new level of wellness in the same old place, and a new level of enjoyment that she brought back with her.

Prepare to have a ball!

It is fun staying healthy the Hawaiian way. As new nourishment courses through your veins and new energy explodes in your day, you will become a new person. Tasks that were burdensome will become challenging. People who were drags will become interesting. Your own personality will become more attractive as your vitality improves.

Life becomes not just more bearable, but a daily celebration.

- Prepare for a greater enjoyment of the food you eat.
- Prepare for a greater enjoyment of your leisure hours.
- Prepare for a greater appreciation of your body.
- Prepare for a greater capacity to work and create.
- Prepare for a greater awareness of beauty.

Living among the Hawaiian people has been full of surprises—delightful ones—for us. Discovering the variety of their music, songs and dances; the depth of their ancient philosophy; the profound love and respect for 'Aina, their land, and appreciation of its awesome beauty; their wisdom about retaining many of the old ways in the face of the increasing pressures of "progress"; and their awareness of the need to preserve their roots.

Today we are all beginning to value these things that seem to run counter to our civilization's headlong rush into an uncertain future. Here in Hawai'i, the clues are still warm leading back to the old ways. And the pace is slower.

Somehow, when the pace is slower, you get just as much done— if not more.

Somehow, when you feel less obligated to duties and responsibilities, you are able to carry them out more effectively.

Somehow, when you are less tense and anxious, there are less reasons for tenseness and anxiety.

These, for us, and for hundreds of thousands of other mainlanders who have either stayed here or brought Hawai'i's ways back with them, are the real health treasures of Hawai'i.

But there are scores of medical treasures to discover, such as the leaf sap that helps burns in an instant (and which you can grow on your balcony or in your kitchen), and the fruit that cleans out arteries that are hardening.

There are scores of body building foods that are as delicious to eat as they are nourishing to the organs.

There are scores of beauty enhancing lotions and potions—all made from vegetation that grows in your area or is obtainable by you.

Roots, herbs, teas, barks, nuts, fruits and vegetables have health secrets that the Hawaiians and Polynesians have discovered and used. Some of them are simply miraculous—that's the only word we can find to describe the dramatic results that we have either heard about or witnessed.

The Hawaiians were such a healthy people, when they were discovered by Captain Cook in the 1700's, that immunities to disease had not been developed. Diseases that were then common in the United States and Europe were not known in the islands. As a result, it took the Hawaiians several generations to adjust to the germs introduced by new settlers and explorers. At one point, measles alone nearly decimated the population.

Hawaiians were then looked upon as a dying race. They seemed to be sickly and prey to any virus that came along. But then their defense mechanisms bounced back and their solid foundation of vitality restored them. They became well-nourished, robust and healthy in stamina and intelligence, and as the late Sir Peter Buck of the Bishop Museum described them, they were "one of the most advanced branches of the Polynesian people." The fact that Buck himself was part Maori from New Zealand added credence to his words.

The Hawaiians were soon joined by some 400,000 laborers for the plantations of sugar cane and pineapple. Recruited with government assistance were roughly 180,000 Japanese and Okinawans, 125,000 from the Philippines, 46,000 Chinese and 17,000 Portuguese from the Azores and Madeira Islands.

Thousands came from Korea, the United States, Puerto Rico, Germany, Russia, Spain and, of course, from the many other islands that dot the Pacific.

Some of these workers later returned to their native countries, but many stayed, thus making the population of Hawai'i a miniature of the earth itself.

These are the people who make up the healthiest population in the world. They come from every culture, every race, every background.

You are no exception. No matter where you live, no matter what your age, sex, religion, race or economic level, you are eligible for the health and advantages enjoyed by this people-conglomerate called the Hawaiians.

All you have to do is discover the health secrets. We wish it had been as easy for us as it is now for you.

KAHUNAS: THE HAWAIIAN MEDICINE MEN

When foreigners began to arrive in Hawai'i, they were quickly integrated into the life and society of the islands. Although each culture maintained its characteristics, the more basic Hawaiian life style was easily assimilated.

Part of that life style consisted in letting a *kahuna* keep you healthy. At the first signs of health trouble, a *kahuna,* the Hawaiian version of the medicine man or wise man, was consulted. He prepared herbs, teas or poultices, and healed his patients with them. But the ingredients used by the *kahunas* were always a well-kept secret.

Only recently have *kahunas* been willing even to talk about their work. The once occult is now being de-occulted. Secret remedies are being made more widely known.

Fortunately for mainlanders, many of the materials used by the *kahunas* are available there. *Kahuna* remedies are disclosed in the pages ahead, where the ingredients or plant material are available to almost everyone.

Some *kahunas* were specialists in herbal healing; others used prayer; still others used massages and other modes of therapy. We have seen many people healed of everything from broken bones to kidney stones by the few *kahunas* who still work their wonders on the islands. But, by and large, the word is out, and what *kahunas* did in secret a hundred years ago are now generally practiced as old-fashioned home remedies.

Take *taro* as an example. This is the potato-like tuber from which the famous *poi* is made. Somehow, the *kahunas* knew that a plaster made of *taro* is the most versatile and penetrating, even more so than mustard.

A *taro* plaster loosens stagnated toxins; draws to the skin surface unwanted oil, fat and mucus; and melts cysts, stones and tumors so that they may be discharged through the skin or elimination system.

This is just one of the many *kahuna* secrets we have collected for your use.

A HAWAIIAN "POTATO" THAT HEALS

We are now going to tell you where to obtain the *taro* and how to prepare a healing poultice or plaster. But first a word about natural cures.

The Federal Center in Disease Control, located in Atlanta, Georgia, is conducting research into the legitimate roles that herbal preparations and other natural remedies can play in meeting the country's health needs. It is part of a larger study of "traditional medicine" going on in 15 other countries, sponsored by the World Health Organization in Geneva, Switzerland.

The reason for this intensified interest in natural remedies has been expressed succinctly by Julian Gold, a scientist at the Atlanta Center, in an interview quoted by the Associated Press: "Two-thirds of the world's population uses traditional medicine for primary care, and if we can't provide health care by conventional medicine, we'll have to find some other way.''

Hawaiians and other Polynesians have always had another way. The arrival of conventional medicine has not displaced this traditional way, but rather it has lived side by side with it.

This is our way of saying that the secrets unveiled in this book are not meant to replace conventional medicine. If you use them, do so in the nature of preventive care and first aid, and continue to use them only under the supervision of your health care specialist.

We are not physicians. We are researchers reporting on substantiated findings, known practices, and traditional customs. We are not offering you a cure for your disease in this book. We are not recommending a treatment for any specific ailment. Rather, we are sharing with you what others have done before and are doing now to successfully treat health problems and also to prevent them.

Now, let's get back to *taro* and its traditional use as a plaster.

Taro, while it is a basic food in Hawai'i, is also common in Japan, West Africa, Puerto Rico and other areas, although it is known by other names. It thrives in swampy soil in wet tropics, growing 2 to 3 feet in height.

You can find the *taro* "potato" year-round in most Oriental and Spanish markets. It is now being stocked by many natural food stores and some supermarkets in large cities.

Select the small, young *taro* for your poultice. Peel off the brown skin. Grate enough of the root for about one-half inch of paste to cover the affected area. If the paste is watery, you may want to add some flour as a binder.

Spread the past on a piece of white cotton cloth and place the cloth over the problem area. If it is a skin-sensitive area, such as the eyelids, you might want to place a piece of extra gauze between the skin and the plaster.

Wear the poultice for about four hours. If there is excessive pain, pressure or throbbing, you may wish to remove it periodically.

The common white potato that you obtain from your supermarket is said to have the same healing properties as the *taro*, but to a lesser degree. Hannah Bond, writing in the August 1978 issue of *East/West Journal*, reports witnessing a nursing mother in Maine draw out a golf-ball-sized cyst from her breast using such a poultice made from Lubek county potatoes.

Mashed *taro* is called *poi,* a Hawaiian food that has contributed greatly to the sturdiness of the Hawaiian people for centuries. (There will be more about the health benefits of this food in Chapter 6.)

MINING FOR HEALTH SECRETS IN POLYNESIA

Hawai'i is the northern apex of a large triangle of Pacific islands generally known as Polynesia. We have visited a number of these islands while conducting our research.

At the western edge lies Fiji, an island where cannibalism was once rampant. At the eastern edge lies Easter Island, where there are still remains of an ancient culture in the form of enigmatic, towering stone faces, but from which the original people have long departed.

At the southern part of this triangle and in the western corner lies New Zealand, abounding in traditional remedies, and with the soil and climate that produce some of the world's most nutritious food. Within the heart of the Polynesian triangle are American Samoa and Western Samoa, where ancient practices flourish; Tonga, the last Polynesian kingdom; and the Cook, Marquesas and Society Islands of French Polynesia.

It will soon be too late to capture for posterity many of the health secrets of these islands. There are many in this book. But the old people are either leaving for other places or dying, and new people are arriving from other places, bringing their own practices with them.

Fortunately, many native health practices are recorded by early explorers and others who have written about the Polynesian cultures. We have been privileged to visit old villages and experience how these beautiful people live and administer to their own health needs.

The late Dr. Paul C. Bragg, self-styled "life-extension specialist," traveled the world over several times in his career of nearly a century as founder of the health food movement in the United States. Polynesia was one of his favorite places. Besides in-depth visits to many of the islands, from New Zealand north, Bragg chose Hawai'i as his home, calling it "the healthiest place on earth."

Every morning, on the beach at Fort DeRussy in Waikiki, nonagenarian Bragg would lead a hundred or more tourists and residents in calisthenics, movements, jogging and swimming, and give a mini-lecture on nutrition. He encouraged dancing, especially the vigorous South Seas dances that he called "the culture of the abdomen."

He challenged his audience—youths and oldsters alike—to look at their bellies and admit how protruding and flabby their organs had become. "We are a nation of constipates!" he would roar. And he would tell his listeners how Polynesian dances and fresh fruits and vegetables help to strengthen and purify the stomach and abdominal area.

You will hear more about Paul Bragg as you read further. He practiced what he preached and taught millions of people to appreciate the kind of natural Polynesian health practices which Hawaiians have been using to live longer.

THE ROLE OF FOOD IN TRADITIONAL HEALTH CARE

The early Polynesians ate fish, game, fruits, nuts, vegetables and tubers. This was a healthful diet.

Cavemen ate cactus, snakes, rabbits, roots, nuts, berries and bark. This, too, was a healthful diet.

Only modern man seems to have introduced the kinds of foods that lead to nutritional problems. Before, the choice was either to starve or to eat. Now, it is either to starve the body by not eating, or to starve the body by eating the wrong kinds of foods. *Or* to eat the right foods and be healthy.

Cavemen, as shown by the research done largely by Vaughn M. Bryant, Jr., associate professor in Anthropology at Texas A & M University, did not have sugar and fat in their diet. Bryant analyzed the "coprolites," or petrified excrement of cavemen found in cliffside caves along the Pecos River valley of southeast Texas. He found evidence of high fiber foods like cactus, low in fat and low in calories.

This follows the same basic composition of Polynesian foods. We will be reviewing these foods in the chapters ahead, from the point of view of their nutritional values as well as their healing properties. But it is probably just as important to stop eating some of the modern refined, chemicalized and prepared foods that our modern diet includes, and to start eating the foods we will be recommending as bursting with life energy and tropical goodness.

Mainlanders who come to live in Hawai'i do not bring with them eating habits that contribute to the high level of health in Hawai'i. They are bringing fast food outlets that popularize pizza, hamburgers and fried chicken. They bring a demand for fast food that encourages supermarkets to move healthier foods aside and make way for canned goods, prepared cereals, packaged cookies, cakes and soft drinks. They bring an insatiable appetite for ice cream, pastries and candies.

Fortunately, the mainland Americans have been in the minority and their total impact has been small. The Japanese are by far the largest segment, and happily the people of Japan have the same high life expectancy as the people of Hawai'i. There is no white sugar or white flour in their food. Instead, there is soybean curd called *tofu*, fish and seaweed—all the kinds of natural foods that are at home in Hawai'i.

Other peoples from Polynesia and the Pacific rim countries have also affected the overall menu of Hawai'i in compatible ways, providing a cosmopolitan restaurant of the Pacific that is like one giant health food restaurant with thousands of choices (all good for you) on its multiracial menu.

The Hawaiian Islands were named the Sandwich Islands by Captain Cook, after the fourth Earl of Sandwich. Only a few years before Cook's voyage, sandwiches had been invented in England and named after this same Earl of Sandwich, so that he could stay at the gambling tables without interruptions for meals. It is well that the name was changed, since at that time sandwiches were unknown in the "Sandwich Islands." The sandwich, especially the kind made of white bread from which all the natural minerals have been removed, is as far removed from the Hawaiian way of healthy living as one can get.

The Hawaiians know how to eat. You will be able to go to your supermarket and buy the same foods that Hawaiians eat, prepared in the Hawaiian way. Whether the influence is Chinese, Japanese, Portuguese or Samoan, the influence on you will be positive—toward a stronger, well-fed body, resistant to disease, free of excess weight and able to manifest more energy than you may have ever known in your life.

THE ROLE OF FOOD AS MEDICINE

Nature has provided us with everything we need to get well and stay well. People who live close to nature "hear" this information. Intuitively, they know what to eat and when.

The American Indian learned nature's lessons well. So did the Hawaiians and other Polynesians.

Take coconut, for example. They knew that this tough nut, with its many layers of protective shell and fibers, was worth the effort to open. They gave coconut meat and coconut milk to thin and emaciated children and adults to build up body tissues and muscles.

If the peanuts whispered about their uses to George Washington Carver, the coconuts fairly shouted about theirs to the Polynesians: "Eat my meat for strength and drink my milk for kidney problems. Let my cream rise and make a health pudding from it. Churn my cream into butter and press the oil from my meat. Use the oil for your skin as a moisturizer, sun protector and conditioner."

These messages of nature became the medical practices of Polynesia. There were no laboratories to create modern antibiotics, but the skin of bananas contain a strong antibiotic. There were no laboratories to prepare digestive aids, but the papaya contains an important digestive enzyme. There were no laboratories to prepare serums to soften arteries, but the pineapple contains an arterial cleanser.

These are nature's lessons that were taught to the Polynesians and handed down from generation to generation, and are now being handed to you between the covers of this book.

- The vegetable mixture that is good for a hangover...
- The leaves that help sores to heal rapidly...
- The substance that helps relieve baby's rashes and is closer than you think...

Scores of remedies and tonics are provided by nature and are indeed used as blueprints in the laboratory. Many are no longer known, as the voice of nature is being drowned out by bulldozers and concrete mixers. Many more are not in this collection because they involve food or plant materials that are not available on the United States mainland.

Those that are included are available to you, some as easily as reaching out for them in the bins and on the shelves of your supermarket. Others may require going to a special store, sending away to a special supplier or locating a particular weed in your back yard or neighborhood.

Follow nature's voice on these pages and your kitchen can become your medicine chest. You can use nature's own remedies, which can frequently be safer and more effective than their laboratory counterparts. But what is even more important, as you follow Polynesian ways, the word "medicine" may drop entirely out of your vocabulary.

INTRODUCTION TO HAWAIIAN AND POLYNESIAN HEALTH SECRETS

We are moving into a time when the specialization of medicine is beginning to reverse itself. The body has been divided into many departments with specialists in each. Now these specialists are beginning to realize that they are dealing with a whole person, in which each part of the body is related to the other.

The old-fashioned general practitioner may be coming back into vogue. The general practitioner may be expanding into a health care specialist who realizes that the whole person does not merely include the body, but also the mind of that person, which really runs the body, and the spiritual and emotional makeup of the person, which really sets the "climate" for mental and physical functioning.

If you talk about this exciting, new, holistic approach to health with a Hawaiian, he will not be impressed. He has known and practiced this approach as far back as he and his forefathers can remember.

You will find that this is not merely a manual of nature's health foods and remedies. It is a holistic health manual.

Hawaiians and other Polynesians used turmeric for skin pimples, *ti* leaves to lower a fever, hibiscus blossom petals to balance their systems and strengthen their babies. But they did much more.

They used a shabby-looking plant which they called the *'uhaloa*, and which we call *Waltheria americana*, for sore throat by peeling the bark off its roots and chewing it for the juice. They used *ualena*, which we know as *Cayenne vervain*, for sprains and broken bones by mashing the leaves with rock salt and rubbing it on the swollen parts four times, morning and night.

Modern Hawaiians and other Polynesians still do these things, and they also eat *poi* as a longevity food, prefer fish as a cholesterol-free protein, and adopt the nutrient-preserving Oriental methods of steam cooking and stir frying. And they do much more, which overflows into the wider horizons of holistic health.

They take long walks. They go on picnics. They swim. They sun. And that is only the beginning.

They dress casually for a special reason. They sing and dance—and it does something to them and for them.

They laugh and have fun. They enjoy *lu'aus* and feasts at the drop of a coconut hat.

They get along with one another. They express *aloha* to the world.

All of this has given the Hawaiians the strength, energy and brimming good health to build a modern state that ranks high in the fields of commerce, social progress and productivity. To visiting mainlanders, it is a paradise. To the people who live here, it is a paradise.

Here, now, is the recipe for paradise.

2

Island Practices That Pay Off Anywhere in Healthful Well-Being

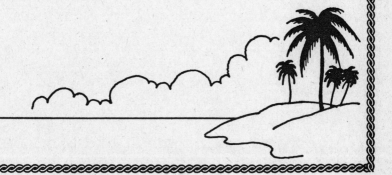

There is so much to health. So many things can go wrong with us and there are so many things to do to keep well.

In order to help you locate information that is of primary concern to you, we are highlighting remedies and practices by specially noting them at the beginnings of relevant paragraphs. We summarize these highlights at the start of each chapter.

As we examine Hawaiian and Polynesian health practices in this chapter from an overall viewpoint, we will begin to zero in on some specific remedies, cures, tonics and preventive practices. These include:

HEALING POULTICE
FAMILY HEALING ROLE
HEALTHFUL "HIGH"
MUSCLE RELAXANT
TOOTHACHE RELIEF
TEA FOR DIABETES
HEALING FOR BURNS
BENEFITS OF GARDENING
GARDENING AS THERAPY
EXERCISE FOR ANY AGE

PROTECTION AGAINST STRESS
BONE STRENGTHENER
LUNG HEALTH
CARDIOVASCULAR HEALTH
NUTRITIOUS MELON
INTERNAL CLEANSER
TREATMENT FOR SORE THROAT
HEALTH TONIC

A woman was walking along a stony beach in Hawai'i. She tripped and fell. A fisherman saw what happened and quickly picked some *limukala,* the common, brown, short-branched seaweed with narrow leaves, usually found wherever seaweed grows.

Helping the woman up, he instructed her to chew the seaweed and place it on the cuts on her face and hands. She did so and reported to him that it took the pain away almost immediately. A few days later, the abrasions healed with no infection.

HEALING POULTICE. In another situation, a young man gashed his arm on a jagged piece of glass. His uncle quickly chewed some of his pipe tobacco and placed it on the wound as a poultice. The bleeding stopped and it healed quickly.

Modern medicine has stopped laughing at so-called primitive medical practices. They are now found to be based largely on valid reasons. When strangers arrived in Hawai'i, they found a people who were remarkably healthy. They had trained doctors, or *kahunas.* Remedies and therapeutic agents were in common use. They observed the personal cleanliness that prevails throughout Polynesia. And they recognized the psychosomatic aspects of illness, long before modern medicine.

FAMILY HEALING ROLE. Serious illness was treated in a holistic way, an approach which modern medicine is only now beginning to respect. A treatment known as *'apu* was used, and is still in use today. It consists of rest, medical treatment, mental relaxation and prayer. The whole family takes part. They abstain from quarreling, entertaining and gossiping. They maintain peace and quiet, and everyone concentrates on the recovery of the ill person.

Douglas S. had a high fever. His wife and two usually vocal children, ages 4 and 7, talked in whispers for two days as Doug drank fruit juice and slept. It was not worry or concern that made them adopt hushed tones, but they were taking part in the treatment. They were "making Daddy well." And Douglas's fever responded by returning to normal at the end of the second day. Not only did the thermometer record the change, but you could hear it in the family's voices.

In the old days, virtually all of the medication prescribed by the *kahuna* came from among 300 varieties of plants and trees on the islands. Mosses, seaweeds and ferns were commonly used. Also used were about ten minerals, including unrefined sea salt and sulphate of soda, which is found in lava fields.

There were specialists among the *kahunas* just as there are specialists among modern doctors today. The *kahuna lapa'au* was the herb specialist. The *kahuna pa'ao'ao* was the pediatrician. The *kahuna haha* was the diagnostician.

The *kahuna haha*, for instance, might administer to a person who had fallen and sustained a head injury by first bringing him a calabash of sea water and a bunch of sugar cane. If, after drinking the water and chewing the cane, the patient vomited, he was considered to be seriously injured with complications to be expected. Today, physicians administer salt with sugar intravenously as an indicator of "delayed shock."

The *kahuna lapa'au* might use powder from the *pia* plant (known by herbalists today as *Leontopetaloides*, and by us as arrowroot) to stop hemorrhaging in the stomach or colon. Today, doctors use a fine powder for this same purpose.

Several doctors have made serious studies of this ancient Hawaiian medical knowledge. F. L. Tabrah, M.D., and B. M. Eveleth, M.D., reporting in the *Hawaii Medical Journal*, say that more of the information has been lost forever than has been handed down through the generations. However, they found many of the secrets among older people living in remote areas of the Big Island, and made a collection of plant medicinals. Unfortunately, most of these materials are not easily available on the mainland and so are not discussed in this book, but the ones that are available will be mentioned in the chapters ahead.

THE DRINK WITH NO HANGOVER

HEALTHFUL "HIGH." One of the natural medicinals that received interest and attention by Drs. Tabrah and Eveleth is *'awa*. This has been and still is a ceremonial drink in Hawai'i and the South Pacific. Sometimes spelled *kawa*, it is a root that causes a pleasant feeling of euphoria with a distinct disinclination to move. The mind remains clear, unlike the effects of alcoholic intoxication. The drinker becomes passive and friendly and is not easily annoyed, again unlike some of the hostile effects of liquor.

The usual *kawa* drink is made from 15 grams of the root stock in a half pint of water. If more than this is imbibed, sleep can ensue. It is a dreamless sleep and the drinker awakes without a hangover, feeling at a high level of well-being.

MUSCLE RELAXANT. Some doctors recommend *kawa* as a nerve sedative. It is also used commercially as a bladder sedative and muscle relaxant. It is available through pharmaceutical houses and herb outlets on the U.S. mainland. It is a muscle relaxant like Valium, but with no side effects. It has been given to astronauts for use prior to reentering the earth's atmosphere.

Kawa exhibits one of the marvels of nature. As much as it is broken down by chemists, its active ingredient cannot be identified. Methystican, kawain, and dihydrokawain—the known active *kawa* ingredients—do not in themselves exhibit the narcotic effects of the whole root extract. So, when the substance is synthesized, the result is not the same.

Traditionally, the whole root extract is prepared for ceremonial drinking by having the root chewed by several of the most attractive young village virgins. It is spit into a calabash, diluted with coconut water and strained.

If you are preparing the *kawa* drink from the root obtained from an herb store—and no village virgins volunteer for the mastication process—the root must be thoroughly pounded in order to produce the proper effects.

There will be more about *kawa*, also known as *'awa*, in Chapter 4.

SOME SECRETS FADE, OTHER SECRETS EMERGE

How we wish we could tell you to go to your drugstore and buy a supply of the *kukui* tree's flowers, nuts and bark, from which the *kahuna lapa'au* could extract numerous effective remedies for asthma, for sores, as a laxative, and for general weakness.

But these are among the secrets that are fading away because of the scarcity of the product. Today, the *kukui* nuts are used for necklaces, but nobody bothers (or remembers how) to prepare the nut oil formerly used to fuel lamps and to provide a protective finish for outrigger canoes, as well as for health purposes.

The white seeds of *mamaki* are still being used for digestive disorders by old Hawaiians, but this plant is scarce even in Hawai'i and soon this, too, will be a legend.

TOOTHACHE RELIEF. There are borderline substances that are available in Hawai'i and other areas of the world, but, for one reason or another, are not generally carried by pharmaceutical or herb outlets. *Puakala,* or Hawaiian poppy, is in this category. Related to the opium poppy, it has been a favorite with Hawaiians for killing pain, both internal and external. When used for a toothache, a piece is cut from the latex-laden root and used as a plug inserted into the offending cavity. Not only does the ache stop, but for some reason not fully understood, that tooth never aches again, suggesting perhaps that the nerves are permanently "put to sleep."

Fortunately, many secrets are being kept alive and the substances that are used are still available, not only in Hawai'i but in other places as well.

TEA FOR DIABETES. Take *hinahina,* for example. It is a plant whose leaves and stems, when dried and made into a tea, are reportedly valuable in fighting diabetes.

Known by botanists as *Artemisia australis,* the *hinahina* plant grows in remote beach areas in many parts of America and other continents. However, because of recent research done on this plant, it is gaining interest with pharmacologists and hopefully will become more generally available.

So the picture is not static. Remedies disappear and reappear. Some are available everywhere; others are difficult to obtain. And this, too, is in flux for specific materials and localities.

Mainlanders have benefited in one particular transition. Centuries ago, Hawaiians used the *'ape* plant for several remedies, but they particularly used the milky sap of the plant *(Alocasia macrorrhiza)* to heal burns.

They would take the *'ape,* cut off a piece of the stalk the size of a forefinger, crush it and mix it with the ashes of half of a burnt coconut. Then they would add one egg white and apply the mixture to the burn.

HEALING FOR BURNS. But then the *aloe* plant was introduced to the islands, where it now grows profusely. It is so easy to use—just cut off the tip of a leaf and apply the sap directly to the burned skin—that *aloe* has supplanted *'ape* as the common island burn remedy.

Aloe is a common houseplant found all over the United States. *'Ape,* on the other hand, is found only in Japan and some other places in Asia, besides in Polynesia where it has been cultivated.

We will talk some more about *aloe* and some of its other healthful uses later.

By and large, the substances we will discuss are all available to you. In some cases, we give specific sources or suppliers because of the special nature of the product.

However, there is much more to Hawaiian health than just these products.

HOW ISLANDERS HAVE FUN TO STAY WELL

Whether you visit Fiji, Samoa, Tahiti or Hawai'i, you will be impressed by the feeling of gaiety among the people.

This very week, while we have been writing these words in Honolulu, there have been two song contests, a cultural festival, a beauty pageant, a parade, a kite-flying contest and a Cherry Blossom Ball.

These kinds of events in other states might go unnoticed by the press and be very poorly attended by the public. However, in Hawai'i they are very important. They are the highlights in the life of the people.

Walter C., a businessman from Seattle, moved here with his family. Once he had been all business; now he is all play. Business comes second. What comes first in Walter's life style are tennis, swimming and socializing. Somehow business gets done, probably just as much as in Seattle. But Walter is enjoying life more here and we see Walter looking younger with each passing year.

There is nothing about having fun in Hawai'i that is exclusive to the islands. You can hold contests in your town, block parties in your neighborhood and lu'aus in your home.

Carole Kai, a well-known local entertainer, got the idea—possibly from the mainland—of holding a bed race as a means of raising money for a charity. In three years it has become a popular event. Participants create make-shift beds on wheels or rollers and race them down a street, one person in the bed and the others pushing.

Bed races can be held anywhere.

Festivals can be held anywhere.

Contests and balls and celebrations can be held anywhere.

All it takes is a relaxed nature. If your board of directors could hold a Wednesday bowling night, profits might go up. If your family could go on a monthly picnic, you might all be closer. If your school PTA could have a covered dish supper annually and put on a humorous show, cooperation between school and parents might improve.

Profits, closeness and cooperation might result, but there is no doubt that the health of all involved will improve. Fun dispels stress.

The need to compete is stressful. The need to get along within a family can be stressful. The need to solve curriculum and other school problems can be stressful. But when you bring into these stressful situations the element of fun, down goes the stress. And up goes everybody's potential longevity.

As you read about the activities of fun-loving Hawaiians, especially as described in Chapters 7, 8, and 9, think in terms of what you can do in your own home and community to have fun, too.

Do not expect that you can have fun with a bed race. It may be the last thing that anybody would want to do where you live. But there must be something else that "fits."

In Laredo, Texas, they hold a hot pepper eating contest once a year, when peppers are harvested. In Wolfsburg, Germany, and its environs, they hold an asparagus festival in the summer when the delicate white asparagus, for which that area is famous, is harvested. A crop, a season, a commemoration—all provide legitimate excuses to have fun.

If people can have fun separately, that's fine. But if, in addition, they also get together for some common purpose of enjoyment, they can have even more fun.

More fun means lower blood pressure, a healthier heart, stronger nerves. These in turn mean more efficient work, greater creativity and productivity, and higher levels of good health.

Hawaiians do not advocate irresponsible fun. There are a small percentage of islanders who shun work and are tropical playboys. There are playboys in every country and state. However, the majority of fun-loving Hawaiians are serious and productive workers.

Whatever your job entails, there is room in your life for fun. We hope you will catch the spirit of Hawaiian fun and that it will become contagious among your friends and co-workers as you introduce a special "medicine" into your life style.

COMMUNAL GARDENING IN HAWAI'I

One of the most healthful pastimes in the United States is grass time. Weeding and mowing the lawn, with one exception, can be a tonic for most people. The one exception is walking behind a power mower that is spewing carbon monoxide fumes.

The people who now live in Hawai'i take advantage of the good weather to manicure their lawns and landscape. It is but one of the many ways in which they stay close to nature. We have seen city folks from San Francisco to New York move to Hawai'i and, where before they never found time to water houseplants, they now get real pleasure in tending their front and back yards. And some go even further. . .

BENEFITS OF GARDENING. Land on the islands is hard to come by. Most houses are on small plots, by United States standards. So public land is used to grow vegetables. A number of the public parks in the center of Honolulu are set aside for folks who want to garden but do not have enough land.

Each person or family is assigned a small plot, usually averaging about 30 by 60 feet. They can plant whatever vegetables or flowers they wish. We have seen beautiful crops of lettuce, string beans, tomatoes, peppers and even some watermelon.

People who live in high-rise apartment buildings frequently plant fruit trees in the narrow patches of grass that are available. When the fruit ripens—whether it is lemons, oranges, grapefruit, guavas or bananas—it's first come, first served (in moderation).

In addition, rural families will add to their available land the sides of roadways and highways. Even though this is state or county land and there is a law against its use for private purposes, officials look the other way and some of Hawai'i's roadsides are bursting with edibles.

Yes, they get "appropriated" from time to time by passersby, but the island people are philosophical about this. They will even offer you samples of what they have grown as a gesture of their *aloha*.

GARDENING AS THERAPY. At least they have benefited themselves by working on the vegetables, enjoying the fresh air, the sunshine and the rapport with nature.

These advantages are not only important for health; they are recognized as important also to restore the will to live in old people, in the mentally ill and in disturbed children.

An important remedy toward the revitalization of the will is rhythmical movement in communion with the beauty of nature, in digging, planting and growing. This is then extended to arts and crafts. Dramatically, the will and heart are revitalized and people young and old, who previously could barely respond to communication, begin to show new interest in themselves and in others.

THE "GREAT OUTDOORS"—ITS REAL MEANING

In the chapters ahead, we are going to describe other Hawaiian outdoor activities. We will mention Sunday running, periodic marathons and daily jogging.

We will mention surfing, sailing and swimming. We will describe a number of beach and water activities, as well as the more inland activities, such as hiking, camping and picnicking. We will describe the special outdoor activities that go on during celebrations and festivals.

Hawai'i is an outdoor place, as are Fiji, New Zealand and Guam. It is easy to go outdoors on any day of the year. Temperatures vary during the day from 75 to 90 degrees Fahrenheit all year round in Honolulu. At night they seldom dip below 60 degrees.

Men can be seen on any day, even in business areas, stripped to the waist. Women wear informal summer attire all year.

When *you* go outside in January, chances are you bundle up. Whether you live in Durham, North Carolina, or Superior, Wisconsin, you think twice about stepping out the front door during winter months. "How cold is it?" "What should I wear?"

So your outdoor sorties during winter months and possibly even much of spring and autumn are made only when necessary.

Most Americans are indoor people. But most Hawaiians and Polynesians are outdoor people. There are good reasons for both ways. But we are going to try to tempt you into becoming more interested in "the great outdoors."

Hothouse varieties of flowers are seldom as vital and lasting as the wild types. Indoor people lack the vitality and possibly even the longevity of outdoor people. We cannot say for sure that every hour you spend outdoors adds two hours or even a half-hour to your life, but we will bet that it will add, not subtract.

By telling you what Hawaiians do to have fun out of doors, we hope it will give you some ideas about what you can do to take advantage of good weather in the city, in the suburbs or in the country—even if it's only walking.

THE MOST EFFICIENT FORM OF EXERCISE

When you are indoors, you sit or stand. When you are outdoors, you move around. Moving around is exercise, and exercise is good for your health.

At a three-day conference on "Exercise in Aging—Its Role in Prevention of Physical Decline," held in October 1977 at the National Institute of Health in Bethesda, Maryland, the following points emerged from the papers presented by researchers from Canada, the United States and Western Europe:

Walking is the most efficient form of exercise.

EXERCISE FOR ANY AGE. Walking can be safely performed as exercise at any age.

PROTECTION AGAINST STRESS. Walking provides a vital reserve which has a protective effect during stress.

About exercise in general, including walking, the conferees agreed:

BONE STRENGTHENER. Exercised bones do not become demineralized and are less likely to break.

LUNG HEALTH. Exercised lungs maintain their capacity longer compared with lungs of sedentary people.

CARDIOVASCULAR HEALTH. Exercised cardiovascular systems show a maximum preservation.

The conferees also talked about the beneficial effects of exercise, like daily walks, on late onset diabetes, which is almost entirely reversed by exercise if you are overweight; about the benefits of exercise in preventing or correcting obesity; about the benefits of exercise in permitting greater food intake and better blood circulation, thus contributing to a higher level of nourishment for all the cells and organs of the body, without risking obesity.

Much to their own surprise, many of the modern researchers found themselves supporting Hippocrates, "the father of medicine," who said over 2000 years ago that walking is man's best medicine.

O'ahu has an excellent bus system. The roads and highways are kept in fine condition. The people travel by bus and car just like people anywhere else. But they also enjoy being outdoors when they are not traveling, and being outdoors means walking.

They hike along mountain trails, but they also stroll along the sidewalk. Men walk with straw hats for protection against the sun. Women often carry parasols. The elderly stroll casually, the young ride skateboards and bicycles or they scamper and dart. They all do what they enjoy doing.

Walking in the great outdoors seems a small price to pay for extended years, if it is indeed a price at all. We will tell you more about how islanders get fun out of their walking and, hopefully, you will see how to adapt their ways to your community and your mainland life style.

THE ONE HAWAIIAN HEALTH INGREDIENT
NOT AVAILABLE TO YOU

As we write this, the sky is a deep blue. The trade winds are blowing gently and distant views are as sharp and crisp as if they were very near. In other words, the air is clean.

There is very little heavy industry in Hawai'i. What smoke there is comes largely from plane and vehicular traffic. Even this pollution is blown out to sea by the almost daily trade winds. Occasionally, the air becomes still. Then a haze begins to become apparent and Honolulu looks like Cleveland, New York, or any other mainland city where pollution is more prevalent.

Hawai'i's air is purified by a vast air conditioning system that stretches over 2000 miles in every direction. When it reaches the island chain, it is purified even more by frequent showers, mostly at night.

There are probably few places in the United States, including Alaska, where the air is as clean as in Hawai'i. Undoubtedly, this clean air contributes to the health of the people who live here.

We cannot deliver this air to you by way of this book, but we can give you ways to take the best advantage of the fresh air wherever you live, based on island principles.

Certainly, being outdoors is one of these. With the exception of standing in the midst of roaring traffic, the air outdoors is fresher than the air indoors. There are ways to make the indoor air fresher, which we will be discussing later, but by definition indoor air has less oxygen and more carbon dioxide and other impurities due to the fact that people gather inside.

We love our Hawaiian air. We hope you will come and experience it some day. But, meanwhile, you can make more of your own fresh air, and help yourself to another ingredient for better health.

WHAT HAWAIIANS AND OTHER POLYNESIANS EAT

This is basically an "eating" book. Yes, we show you many ways that islanders stay healthy and scores of remedies for different ailments, but every day they eat in a special way that keeps them slender and healthy, and this is perhaps the biggest Hawaiian and Polynesian health secret of all.

It all started centuries ago when the islanders subsisted largely on *taro*, yam, breadfruit, bananas, coconut, sweet potato and fish.

They also hunted jungle fowl, wild ducks and geese, and caught the *kolea*, or plover, by imitating its whistle.

Today, different cultures have introduced new foods as they arrived from Japan, China, the Philippines and other Pacific rim countries. But fresh fruit, fresh vegetables, fish and poultry still dominate the diet.

Ancient Hawaiians were experts at aquaculture. They built and stocked fish ponds in bays and inlets. These were a constant source of choice mullet and other tasty fish.

Today, the fish ponds are still there, but without any fish. Some are silted, partially filled in, or have been converted to marinas. Instead, new aquaculture methods are being used to raise oysters, catfish and prawns. And boats go out to sea to bring in an endless variety of ocean fish, when the waters are not too rough.

Fish is such a popular and universally enjoyed food by all the diverse cultures here that it is practically always in short supply. On certain holidays, it is not turkey that goes up in price, but fish. During the past year, it hit $7.00 and $8.00 a pound on more than one occasion.

Thanks to mass marketing methods and modern distribution, fish is probably more available to you than to Hawaiians who live surrounded by the ocean. Fish is a prime health food in the islands, one which you can enjoy economically and frequently, no matter where you live.

So are fruits and vegetables, and we will be discussing the best of these and why they are so good for you.

Hawaiians and other Polynesians have not taken to fatty meats and rich pastries. They have not adopted prepared foods from the mainland as readily as they have been brought here by those who move to Hawai'i from the mainland. Synthetic and "glued-together" foods make little headway here. Yes, the same products you see in your supermarkets are on the shelves here, too, but they are not the staples. The staples are the fresh produce.

Hawaiians know about TV dinners that need only to be heated in the oven, canned dinners that need only to be warmed up, prepared dough that turns into rolls in the oven, synthetic cheeses, and pies and snacks that need only to be unwrapped.

But most natives leave these processed foods for the visitors and new mainland residents, and instead they buy more natural products.

Chemicals and additives, which form the "glue" that holds these foods together and causes them to last longer on the shelves, are not exactly longevity ingredients. Although most of these substances are harmless, several have been linked to serious and even fatal diseases. Many others among the 2500 food additives being used on the mainland today are causing health problems without our being aware of it.

As the pace of life quickens on the islands, the longevity rate may decrease. If it does, a good part of the reason will be a tendency to adopt quick and easy foods prepared by man rather than by nature—foods with preservatives, anti-oxidants, stabilizers, thickeners, leavening agents, maturing and bleaching agents, curing agents, emulsifiers, sweeteners, flavors, colors, anti-caking and foaming agents.

These are foods robbed of nutritional value and endowed with potential irritants and pollutants. They were not part of anyone's fare 100 years ago and have been resisted more successfully by islanders than by mainlanders, giving islanders a positive health advantage.

ISLANDERS MAKE HEALTH MISTAKES, TOO

Islanders have natural instincts that come through loud and clear for them because they live closer to nature than most mainlanders.

When Captain James Cook introduced watermelon to Hawai'i by leaving seeds here in 1779, the native Hawaiians kept it growing and going, recognizing in it a nutritious food. The watermelons grown in Hawai'i are smaller than those on the mainland and the skin is thinner. They have a long growing season, centering on May through September but often preceding and extending this by a month or two.

NUTRITIOUS MELON. The Hawaiians had no way of knowing scientifically that watermelon is good for you; that an average wedge is relatively low in calories, having no more than a medium-sized apple or pear; that it provides half of our minimum daily requirements of vitamins A and C; and that it is a source of calcium, phosphorus and iron.

INTERNAL CLEANSER. Yet, they created a place for watermelon in their natural storehouse of remedies and today watermelon is still used as a cleansing agent. Eaten at least four hours after a heavy meal, it acts to purify the system of residual toxins and to flush the kidneys.

More recently, however, Hawaiian intuitive perception of what is good and what is not good appears to have lost its sharpness. An example is fruit juices.

The juice of Hawaiian fruit is the elixir of life. When we came here as tourists nearly 20 years ago, we reached for fruit juice on the supermarket shelves. To our dismay, all we could find were fruit "nectars" and fruit "drinks." There was passion fruit, guava fruit and papaya—separate, combined or mixed with orange—but only in sugared form.

Guava nectar is still today only 15 percent guava juice. And the "drinks" have as little as 10 percent fruit juice. The rest is sugar and water.

So hypnotized by this sugared variety have the Hawaiian taste buds become that now they consider it to be the real thing. Visitors sample it for breakfast but it is too sweet even for mainland tastes.

Recently, one of the two large producers of these sugared fruit drinks introduced the frozen variety to California markets. It was a flop.

"Too much sugar," complained the California shoppers as they passed up second purchases of the papaya nectar and guava nectar and "passo-guava" combination nectar.

Recently, the supplier found what may be the answer—mixing these juices with the only Hawaiian fruit juice that demands no sugar—pineapple. Even if this is found to be palatable on the mainland,

Hawaiians will still go on buying the sweetened variety and adding unneeded sugar to otherwise wholesome fruit juice.

This is the one glaring departure from natural health practices that we have seen here. Maybe it has something to do with sugar cane being a major crop in Hawai'i—a sort of local patriotism. Maybe not. Suffice it to say that, because Hawaiians do many more things right than they do wrong, we can forgive them for this one transgression.

THE PACIFIC BASIN AS A MEDICINE CHEST

As we glean health secrets from the Hawaiians, we tap many cultures. Sitting out in the middle of the Pacific Ocean, Hawai'i has been the meeting place of East and West. O'ahu, the name of the island on which Honolulu sits, means "the gathering place." It was so named because people from neighboring islands of Maui, Lana'i, Moloka'i, Hawai'i (the Big Island), Kaua'i, and Ni'ihau were frequent visitors.

Now the name is even more appropriate as people gather there from Japan, China, Korea and the Philippines on the west; Samoa, Tahiti, Tonga, Fiji, New Zealand and the Marquesas on the south; and the countries of North and South America to the east.

All bring with them the necessities of their own life styles and health is a basic ingredient of each.

Recently, the University of California at Los Angeles held a symposium on "Popular Dimensions of Brazil." Featured was the Brazilian system known as "cura." As late as 1973, 60,000,000 Brazilians were using cura, which means curing. They were slipping out of hospitals to visit healers for cura treatment, and supplementing their physicians' prescriptions with cura.

What is cura? It is both psychological and spiritual treatment. One speaker from a Texas university described cura as similar to the principle upon which the World Health Organization (WHO) functions, namely that health is a state of complete physical, mental and social well-being, and not merely the absence of infirmity or disease.

WHO is urging the maximum use of folk medicines in reaching its goal of providing health care for all the people of the world by the year 2000.

After listening to the speakers on Brazil's popular medicine, one conferee—historian David Sweet—called it a "vibrant strategy" and a "people's therapy."

This is also a good way to describe the Hawaiian and Polynesian health system. It is vibrant, holistic and communal.

TREATMENT FOR SORE THROAT. Yes, it is fine to copy the Samoans and use the bark of the mango tree—boiling it and gargling the essence—as a treatment for sore throat.

HEALTH TONIC. Yes, it is fine to use the Tongan's secret of taking the sap of the ironwood tree as a health tonic.

Yes, all of these remedies—and we will be providing you with scores—have a longstanding record of effectiveness.

But, the Hawaiian and Polynesian *cura* involves staying well as much as it involves healing disease. It means a total program of physical, mental and spiritual health. It's dynamic. It's complete. It works.

Now let's get into it.

3

Secrets of Hawaiian Healing Herbs and Roots

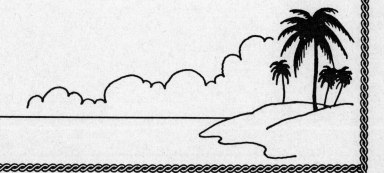

In this chapter, we mine for remedies along the streets and lanes of old Hawai'i as well as in the valleys and the hills. Polynesian cures are intermingled with those of the Japanese, Chinese and Filipinos in this meeting place of the Pacific.

In the process, we discover natural remedies for the following disorders:

FEVER	BURNS
RHEUMATIC PAIN	WEAKNESS
ASTHMA	TUBERCULOSIS
POSTPARTUM PROBLEMS	FEVER FLUSHES
NASAL CONGESTION	LOWERED RESISTANCE
COUGH	SEXUAL PROBLEMS
CUTS	DEBILITY
CONSTIPATION	IMPOTENCY
DIABETES	SINUS
SORE THROAT	LOW ENERGY
FESTERING WOUND	INTERNAL HEMORRHAGING
BOILS	DYSENTERY
PILES	HIGH BLOOD PRESSURE
TOXICITY	INSECT BITES
BAD BREATH	SUNBURN
PIMPLES	BLISTERS

ULCERS   *CIRCULATORY PROBLEMS*
SKIN PROBLEMS   *OPEN SORES*
INFANT CONSTIPATION   *CATARACT*
NURSING PROBLEMS   *ARTERIOSCLEROSIS*
CATARRH   *HIVES*
STOMACH DISTRESS   *BLEEDING*
PAIN   *MEASLES*
CARDIAC PROBLEMS

Legend has it that Lonopuha, an ancient chief on the western side of the Big Island, had a reputation of having never been hurt or sick. A passing stranger, hearing of this, said, "He will be hurt and he will be sick."

Almost immediately, Lonopuha accidentally jabbed his foot with a gardening tool. Bleeding was profuse and he fainted. Someone remembered what the stranger had said and hurried after him. The stranger introduced himself as Kamaka, the god of healing. He hurried back, on the way gathering leaves and fruit from *popolo* bushes (not available on the mainland) and calling for sea salt. When he reached Lonopuha, he pounded the leaves, fruit and salt together to make a poultice for the foot wound.

The poultice worked and Lonopuha recovered. He implored Kamaka to teach him the art of healing with herbs. Kamaka agreed. The Kamaka-Lonopuha school of medicine, using herbs and prayer, became the source of herbal treatments still used in Hawai'i today.

Their validity may now be confirmed by cross-referencing these herbal treatments with those of other countries and cultures, where they are frequently found to be in use for the same problems.

A TREE LEAF WITH HEALING POWERS

The eucalyptus tree is indigenous to the islands of the South Pacific. Its many varieties, including a number of shrubs, have spread to New Zealand and Australia, and some 200 varieties have been introduced into California, where it is continuing to spread.

Wherever the eucalyptus trees and shrubs grow, the distillate made from the leaves is used as both an antiseptic and a vapor inhalant for some respiratory diseases.

Eucalyptus oil is now obtainable in most pharmacies. Your pharmacist can tell you about its most common uses and give you directions.

FEVER. Hawaiians call eucalyptus *pale-piwa*, which literally means "ward off fever." It was used in a steam bath. A few drops of the oil in the water that is turned into steam at your local Turkish bath would come closest to the Hawaiian method of a sweat bath. But now some people derive fever-reducing benefit by taking a hot bath with a few drops of oil in the tub water.

RHEUMATIC PAIN. These baths are also said to alleviate rheumatic pain. Again, a few drops of eucalyptus oil are placed in the hot bath water. It is not generally known just how the oil does its work, but it is a penetrant and must find its way to where its antiseptic and healing qualities may be put to use.

ASTHMA. It is also a vaporant. Its healing factors can be inhaled, benefiting the respiratory tract. In New Zealand, the leaves are placed in steaming hot water and the vapor is inhaled to relieve asthma. Of course, the oil can be used instead of the leaves.

POSTPARTUM PROBLEMS. New Zealanders also find that a bath with the leaves immersed in the bath water helps new mothers with postpartum recovery. Again, the oil can be substituted for the leaves.

NASAL CONGESTION; COUGH. David B. had a bad cold. His nose was so stuffed that he could hardly breathe, and he had developed a cough that produced a volume of mucus. He remembered that his parents used eucalyptus leaves when he was a child by placing them in a steaming kettle.

Using the oil instead, David made himself comfortable by the kitchen range and waited for the kettle, containing the few drops of oil in water, to boil.

With a towel over his head to capture the fumes, he then began to breathe the mixture of steam and air. In a minute or two, he noticed a clearing of his nasal passages. He kept up the process for about five minutes. He found that his cough was less frequent. In two days, doing this twice a day, he was back to normal.

COMMON WEEDS THAT ARE GOOD MEDICINE

CUTS. Bob F. cut his head on a protruding cabinet door. His grandmother hastened outside and picked some *honohono* grass, known as "Wandering Jew" on the mainland. She squeezed out the sap or juice and applied it directly to the cut on his head. The bleeding stopped and the injury healed quickly.

"Wandering Jew" is a weed. If you had it in your garden, you might pull it up and throw it out, but some people value it as a houseplant.

There are a number of common weeds that are used in Hawai'i and Polynesia as remedies with remarkable success.

CONSTIPATION. Plantain is a weed that, when made into a tea, acts as a mild laxative. We will show you more uses of this weed in the next chapter. But you would never expect this common weed to provide relief for what the medical professional calls an incurable disease: diabetes.

DIABETES. Jack P. had severe diabetes. According to his doctor, his sugar count was over 300 and he needed hospital care. When Jack told this to one of the tenants in his building, she said, "I want to fix something for you."

She picked plantain from the curbside and dried the leaves in a shady spot. She then mixed the leaves in a blender to make small bits of them and simmered one tablespoon of these in four cups of water for an hour.

Jack's instructions were to drink about a cup of this liquid once a day. A few weeks later, he returned to see the doctor. To the doctor's amazement, Jack's sugar count was down to 70.

Common weeds that are one man's nuisance may be another man's cure.

SORE THROAT. One old-timer who is still interested in teaching the old ways chews the leaves of the *Waltheria americana,* a common mainland weed, to relieve sore throat.

FESTERING WOUNDS; BOILS. The New Zealand Maoris use plantain to heal festering wounds and boils. They first draw blood from the wound. Then they heat the leaves and place them face down on the wound to draw out pus and poisons.

PILES. They also use this common weed to cure piles. They make a concentrated tea from it and use it in one of two ways. They either sit in the hot liquid or squat over the steaming tea. By "coincidence," the ancient Greeks also used plantain to cure piles.

The Maoris use another common mainland American weed known as "lamb's quarters" as a cure for boils. So they certainly have a respect for the healing qualities of weeds.

COMMON HERBS WITH UNCOMMON USES

Mint is grown by many families all over the mainland, even in kitchens. It is used to flavor iced tea, to make hot tea, as a garnish in fruit salad and in a score of common recipes.

TOXICITY. But few people on the mainland know that it is an effective perspirant. Two cups of mint tea drunk as hot as possible induces perspiration to get rid of body poisons, according to the Maoris of New Zealand and other Polynesian areas.

BAD BREATH. The rose is a beautiful shrub. Wild roses are admired wherever they grow and they grow practically everywhere on the mainland. But few admirers of the rose realize that the leaf is chewed by many in Polynesia to sweeten breath.

PIMPLES; BURNS. Also, when the leaves are boiled in water or just soaked in water for several days, the resulting potion is known to get rid of pimples and heal burns. Yes, look at the beauty of rose blossoms, but see in the leaves that surround these blossoms one of nature's many herbal remedies.

WEAKNESS. No one seems able to recall when parsley was introduced to the islands, but you will often see more than a sprig put on plates as a garnish. That is because its value is recognized functionally as well as esthetically. Parsley's function is to supply iron, vitamin C and iodine, but islanders eat it without this chemical analysis, knowing intuitively that it is a body builder and blood purifier.

THE HAWAIIAN SYSTEM OF HERBAL CURES

So complete was the Hawaiian knowledge of herbal cures and remedies that complicated combinations of herbs were often prepared in special ways that nobody could possibly duplicate today.

It would be of little value to you if we gave you the following procedure for preparing an herbal blood purifier extracted from the way it was originally published some 50 years ago:

> *Take eight pieces of the root hibiscus; four pieces of the Bobea bark the size of the palm of the hand; the same amount of mountain-apple bark; the bark of eight Waltheria americana roots; one Desmodium uncinatum plant without the burrs . . . two pieces of tree fern that are partly dried . . . four Morinda citrifolia fruits; a segment and a half of red sugar-cane.*
>
> *Thoroughly pound together. Put into a container having about a quart of water. Cook with six red-hot stones. Empty into the fibers of the Cyperus laevigata. The patient then takes a mouthful of the liquid three times a day before meals, for five successive days.*

Little wonder that you and I would rather buy a drugstore tonic!

Today, few Hawaiians go through the process followed by their forefathers, and the prepared herb teas that are available on supermarket shelves and in health food stores are their preference.

ASTHMA; TUBERCULOSIS. Still, a fisherman on the beach tells us that his family and friends use common clover as a cure for asthma. You pull up the entire clover root ball, clean it, pound it with a small piece of sugar cane, sprinkle a small amount of red earth as you would pepper, strain, heat with water and drink. He knows of people who have also used this successfully for tuberculosis.

We frequently see similarities between the American Indian medicine man's system and the Hawaiian one. An intuitive approach to diagnosis is commonly used. A Hopi medicine man has explained to us how, after examination of a patient, he goes out into the hills and waits. He is then "moved" or prompted to pick certain leaves, herbs or roots. He returns, prepares a poultice or tea, and the patient recovers.

Old folks, not necessarily native Hawaiians, do the same here. Edwin S., who moved here from the Midwest, and who worked in a high pressure job, found that he would suffer unaccountably for days with a high fever. His skin even broke out in a heat-like rash. His doctor could find no cause.

FEVER FLUSHES. Ed married a Filipino woman and, one day when he had one of his attacks of fever, she went out into their garden and picked a few handfuls of lemon leaves and guava leaves. She let them simmer in hot water for 45 minutes. She then prepared the tub for a hot bath, strained out the leaves and poured the liquid into the tub water. After the bath, Ed felt better, his fever was down, the rash disappeared and up until now he has not been troubled at all by those fevers.

Undoubtedly, the Filipino woman was remembering something from the distant past or hearsay. But she was also exhibiting a profound faith in nature.

Scientists are finding out that faith and expectation are powerful healers. They are forced to examine what the human mind can do. It is now suspected by some that because important elements in human nutrition sit side by side on the periodic table of elements—meaning that only one electron spells the difference—the mind might have the ability to move that electron and change, for example, magnesium to potassium, whenever one is ingested and the other is in short supply.

Certainly, the ability of the mind to detect intuitively what the body needs is not in question. Even before the scientific acceptance of psychic functioning, scientists were well aware of the attraction of animals to the very types of grasses, weeds or herbs that were needed by them to rectify disease.

There is no doubt that this type of psychic or intuitive functioning played a part in the establishment of the Hawaiian system. It not only cut short the long periods of trial and error, but led to the complicated combinations, such as the one described above, that proved eminently effective for them.

George Washington Carver claimed over 50 years ago that the peanuts "talked" to him and told him about the many uses to which that previously unpopular crop could be put. Did the wormwood weed "speak" to the American Indian, too, and say, "I relieve stomach disorders when drunk as a tea"? Did the horehound weed say, "I relieve colds"? Did the globe thistle say, "Boil me, mash me and put me on a wound, and I will stop pain, draw out impurities and eliminate swelling"?

By word of mouth, by quiet wisdom, by trial and error, somehow nature gets the message through to us. And despite the roar of civilization, her voice is still heard. We have heard it and now you are hearing it.

The Hawaiian and Polynesian herbal cure systems have their roots exactly where the American Indian roots are and, in fact, exactly where other ancient cultures that still survive have their roots.

The only reason for the differences is in the environment, the varieties of plant life that exist in a particular place.

Wherever one lives, there is a natural remedy to be found. By remedy is meant a substance that alters bodily functions so that the body mobilizes to cure itself.

FIVE ROOTS THAT WORK HEALTH MAGIC

Herbs, taken from above the ground, seem to mobilize corrections to injury or malfunction.

Roots, taken from below the ground, seem to mobilize reinforcement to energy, stamina and health.

Ginger has been around for a long while. The first European to have seen a live ginger plant is said to have been Marco Polo, while he was visiting the kingdom of Genghis Khan in the late thirteenth century. But ginger root was known in England earlier than this, being as common in English trade as pepper.

LOWERED RESISTANCE. Ginger developed an enviable reputation as a builder of energy, stamina and resistance to disease. King Henry VIII of England recommended that it be taken with wine and herbs as a preventive to the dreaded plague that was periodically devastating Europe.

SEXUAL PROBLEMS; DEBILITY. Ginger has and is being used to build up virility in men and desire in women. It is also said to prolong life.

Ginger is a favorite in Hawai'i. You might see fresh ginger occasionally in supermarkets on the mainland, but it is always in abundant supply in Hawai'i. Here it is a recognized source of health. We will say more about ginger in the next chapter.

Another root that was recognized by the Chinese centuries ago for its life support qualities is *ginseng*. *Ginseng* is now extinct in China but recent reports indicate that its cultivation may be under way. It is already being cultivated in Korea. However, in the United States it grows wild, although it is scarce, in about half the states.

IMPOTENCY. Like the root of the ginger plant, *ginseng* root is valued for its effect on male potency. Chewed or drunk as a tea, it also is used to extend life when death threatens. There will be more about *ginseng*, too, in the next chapter.

Both *ginseng* and ginger are valued in Hawai'i, largely because of the "missionary" work done for these health builders by the Chinese segment of the population.

It is valued as a food for the same characteristics that it exhibits as a live plant.

SINUS. Lotus is another therapeutic root. One of its most popular current uses is for sinus. Grate fresh lotus root and add flour to make a paste. Apply it to the lower forehead and around the eyes for a few nights upon retiring. Mucus discharged through the nose then leads to a clearing of the sinus.

The *kuzu* plant is a climbing vine that flourishes throughout most of Japan's mountain wilderness. It grows so thickly that it converts forests into impenetrable jungles. Its root is as dauntless as its vine. It will grow straight into mountainsides, sometimes to a depth of several feet, and has been known to pierce bedrock.

The vine of the *kuzu* plant is used as rope to tie house rafters together. Almost unbreakable, it can weather for years. The *kuzu* grows in the United States, too, especially in Georgia, where it is considered a pesky weed.

LOW ENERGY; WEAKNESS. The root of the *kuzu* plant is used to make a clean, chalk-like starch that turns translucent when cooked. Although similar in appearance to arrowroot and often confused with it, it is quite a different food and one which we hear about repeatedly as a source of energy and abounding strength.

The foodstuff called *kuzu* is the nutritional essence of the hardy plant. Among the heaviest and most concentrated of starches, it contains more calories per gram than honey. However, honey is a quick burning sugar, while *kuzu* is slow burning. It is a long sustaining source of energy, unmatched by other starches. In addition, it takes only a small fraction of the energy it generates for its own digestion as it is absorbed quickly and readily by our digestive metabolism.

Seen under a microscope, the starch of *kuzu* forms small five-sided crystals. In comparison with other starches, such as potato starch, it is minute. The globules of potato starch are 10 to 20 times larger and do not crystallize.

Some 350 kilotons of *kuzu* are processed in Japan each year, most of it by one family that has been in business for over 100 years. The processing method is another plus for its use as a health booster. No chemicals or preservatives are added and only fresh mountain water is used.

Repeated washing of the crude starch is required and this can be done only in the cold of winter when the enzymes used in the process are less active, which can otherwise adversely affect the quality of the starch.

You can get *kuzu* at Oriental food stores and in some health food stores. Use it instead of cornstarch or arrowroot.

Dilute it first in water. Heat over a low flame, stirring constantly, until its milk-white color becomes suddenly translucent. It makes an excellent thickener for soups and sauces. But, more important, it is another reason why the people of Hawai'i are among the healthiest in the world. See yourself acquiring the energy and strength of the *kuzu* vine and root as you enjoy it with your meal.

Special note: We said above that *kuzu* can be used instead of arrowroot. As a starch, we vote *kuzu* as the more healthful. But arrowroot is no slouch. It deserves a place in your kitchen, instead of the more common and less nutritious starches. The starch of arrowroot was used by American Indians to draw out the poison from an arrow wound, hence its name. It is used more commonly in health-conscious Hawai'i than in most areas of the U.S. mainland.

INTERNAL HEMORRHAGING; DYSENTERY. Starch made from roots, according to the people of Hawai'i, is *"no ka oi"* (the best)! Arrowroot *(pia)* goes back perhaps thousands of years in its use by Polynesians. The arrowroot starch was mixed with water in various strengths and taken internally to stop hemorrhaging in the stomach or intestines. Five times a day was the recommended frequency. It was also used in the same manner to stop dysentery.

Arrowroot, compared with a substance like cornstarch, is an elixir. Cornstarch has three times the calories per unit weight and these are empty calories—empty of fiber; empty of calcium, phosphorus, potassium and iron; empty of vitamin C and B. Arrowroot has all of these minerals and vitamins in significant amounts.

Proof again that the starch of the root is the starch to use.

A PLANT WITH EXTERNAL AND
INTERNAL HEALING PROPERTIES

HIGH BLOOD PRESSURE. A truck driver in Honolulu is overweight and has high blood pressure. His doctor wants him to lose weight and take certain medication. This man likes his food too well, though, and also has his own ideas about medication for lowering blood pressure. So, a few hours before each visit to the doctor, he takes *aloe* juice made by squeezing the sap from the tip of an *aloe* plant leaf into some water.

"Not bad," says the doctor when he measures his blood pressure, and gives him another reprieve.

Aloe is a cactus-like plant which, as we mentioned earlier, is grown indoors and outdoors throughout the United States. However, most people look upon it as easy to grow and decorative, not as the amazing internal and external healer that it is.

BURNS. The *Aloe vera* is mentioned in the Bible a number of times. But science has largely ignored it until recently when it was adopted for use in a number of burn centers.

INSECT BITES; SUNBURN; BLISTERS. *Aloe* sap helps kitchen burns almost instantly. It takes the sting and itch out of insect bites. Spread the jelly-like substance on sunburns and on blisters for relief.

ULCERS. Betty S., who runs a dress shop in a fashionable Waikiki hotel, drank *aloe* in water for her ulcers. It proved successful and she now bottles it as a sideline, talking it up among her customers.

If you cannot find an *aloe* plant in your local nursery, perhaps a neighbor has one and can spare part of it for you to plant. They grow quite prolifically and even daily use does not seem to halt the plant's ability to restore itself—and then some.

SKIN PROBLEMS. *Aloe* is now finding its way into skin care creams with therapeutic properties. Ideal, Inc. of Dallas, Texas, is an international marketing company that handles health related products and is currently distributing *aloe* creams direct to the consumer.

THE FLOWER THAT LIKES YOU

A mother picks hibiscus blossoms and chews them. She then places the chewed petals in her infant's mouth and the baby swallows them.

INFANT CONSTIPATION. This unusual baby food is often administered as early as seven days after birth, especially when the baby's normal bowel movements are erratic.

There are two main varieties of hibiscus, one providing a red flower, the other yellow. They grow in southern states and are frequently used as a decorative hedge. Both are said to have the same medicinal value.

NURSING PROBLEMS. When a new mother eats the red-pink hibiscus flower, she produces a plentiful supply of milk for her infant.

Some tropical countries are now realizing that one variety of the bountiful hibiscus is a nutritious vegetable, and it is becoming an exportable item.

DEBILITY; CONSTIPATION. In Hawai'i, those "in the know" chew not only on the petals and flower buds but the leaves as well. The slimy juice is deemed a tonic for a run-down condition or debility as well as a gentle laxative. It apparently works by softening the contents of the intestines and colon.

CATARRH. Health food stores carry hibiscus tea. It is said to be helpful for chronic catarrh.

It is said that when a Hawaiian lass wears a hibiscus in her hair, on the right side it means she's "tooken," on the left side she's "lookin'," and in the middle she's "tooken, but still lookin'." It could also mean that she is carrying her tonic with her and will later eat it.

THE HIDDEN CURATIVE POWERS IN FOOD

"What in the world is that?" we asked the mother of a Filipino friend of ours who was sitting in the kitchen drinking a jet-black brew.

"It's for my stomach," grimaced the lady, "I ate too many *malassadas.*"

Malassadas are the Portuguese version of the doughnut.

STOMACH DISTRESS. She explained how her parents and their parents before them had always found relief from stomach distress by putting dry rice in a heavy pan and roasting it over a high burner. Stir the rice until it becomes quite black. Then pour boiling water over it, strain and drink.

It is called rice coffee and no sooner had she finished the cup, than she was enjoying obvious relief from the distress.

COUGH. Lana J., formerly of Los Angeles, had a persistent cough. It had plagued her for over a week. She was leery of cough medicines and their sedation ingredients. Her Hawaiian boyfriend told her about a watercress cure. She put watercress through her juicer. Then she mixed it with enough water to make it palatable.

She drank the mixture three times that day. When she awoke the next day, the cough was gone.

The practitioners of allopathic medicine have a difficult time accepting such cause-and-effect relationships. Analyze a cup of watercress and you come up with water, fiber, 0.9 grams of protein, 27 milligrams of vitamin C, 547 International Units of vitamin A, some calcium, some carbohydrate, etc., but no special chemical or ingredient that might be helpful to coughs.

Analyze *ginseng* and you find potassium, phosphorus, magnesium, calcium, sodium, aluminum, iron, silicone, barium, stratium, titanium, manganese, glucose and volatile oils. But nothing special or uncommon.

Analyze ginger, arrowroot and other roots and herbs and you come up with beneficial minerals but not in quantities that offer logical reasons for the root or herb to be of medicinal value.

Louise A. brought her mother here when she came from New York City. Now at 82, her mother had a constriction in her digestive system and could not hold down her food. The doctors refused to operate because of her advanced age. Louise knew a Hawaiian *lomi* masseur. He agreed to work on her mother. He massaged her stomach and body for five days, hours at a time. At the end of the fifth day, her mother was able to eat again.

Here, perhaps, is an analogy of how nature works through roots and herbs. Internal actions of glands and organs are stimulated by different herbs and roots. It is not an outside agent that does the healing work, but rather the body's own healing ability that is somehow stimulated.

"Somehow" is the clinker that jams the logical thought processes of the chemist. Until "somehow" is seen under a microscope, it is not accepted scientifically.

But nature does not stand on ceremony. Accepted or not, the roots and herbs work for man and for animals. Her secret ingredients remain secret, and the world divides into two parts—those who first insist on knowing the secret, and those who just accept her healings without question.

COMMON HERBS AND THEIR MEDICINAL USES

The Chinese have had a profound influence on health in Hawai'i. Chinese restaurants, herb stores and medical practitioners far exceed the proportion that the Chinese population represents to the total.

Whereas the people of Hawaiian blood seem to be shifting away from the old methods, the Chinese are actively perpetuating their ancient cures here. One example is acupuncture. There are so many acupuncturists in Hawai'i that they have a licensing and regulating committee at the state government level, just as do doctors, dentists, psychologists and other professional groups.

We would like to list some common herbs used by people in Hawai'i today, largely traceable to Chinese origin. Because of the length of time that these herbs have been in use, the exact method of use has branched out. Some use an herb as a poultice for a length of time, others use the same herb for the same condition, but iron the herb or press it down with a hot water bottle.

It would be presumptuous of us to say how much of an herb should be used and how it should be applied or ingested, as each herb seems to work its wonders despite many different ways of applying it.

The old physicians laid great value on herb mixtures and private ways of applying them. Some of these were jealously guarded as family secrets and handed down from generation to generation as family legacies.

Many of these application methods included instructions regarding the time of day and phases of the moon. These are now largely disregarded but new biological research is lending credence to these factors as the biological rhythms of life processes are becoming more fully understood.

Although there are many herb teas for internal use, many herbs are administered externally. There are several external methods. One is to inhale the fumes from a brew. There is the bath treatment where an extract of the herb, made by boiling, is placed in the bath water. Then there is the poultice or plaster method where the herb is mashed or powdered, made into an ointment and spread on the affected part.

Because of the diversity of ideas as to which is the best way to apply an herbal remedy, we list some here and their basic medical use without detailed instructions. We suggest external use unless otherwise stated. We also suggest that you try small amounts to test the results before going further with either external or internal use.

Disorder	Herb (common name)	Use
PAIN	Aconite (a flowering bulb)	External
WEAKNESS	Sesame	Tea
	Magnolia	Tea
CARDIAC AND	Camphor	Inhalant
CIRCULATORY	Mint	Tea
OPEN SORES	Plantain	External
	Gardenia	External
TOXICITY	Garlic	Internal
	Hibiscus	Internal
	Shrubby horsetail	Tea
	Dandelion	Tea
ASTHMA	Mugwort	Tea
	Angelica	Tea
	Mulberry leaves	Tea
	Sesame	Tea
CATARACT	Ginger	External
	Maidenhair leaves	External
ARTERIOSCLEROSIS	Aloe	Internal
COUGH	Angelica	Tea

MORE REMEDIES FROM THE PAST

The Hawaiians called it *'uhaloa*. The pharmaceutical houses call it *Waltheria americana*. Its roots were chewed to relieve sore throat.

HIVES; BLEEDING. The Hawaiians called it *honohono*. The pharmaceutical houses call it *Commelina diffusa*. Its sap was used as an astringent for hives and as a blood coagulant for lacerations.

MEASLES. When foreigners arrived and introduced measles, for which the Hawaiians had developed no immunity, *honohono* was found to relieve the measle rash.

To break the measles, the *kahunas* used pepper and dried fruit boiled in a lobster shell. It seemed to work by inducing fever and breaking the measle attack.

And, finally, the Hawaiians called this herb *pala'a*. We call it lace fern *(Sphenomeris chusana)*. By any name, when drunk as a tea, it softens stools and relieves constipation.

Again—a warning—some of these plants may contain substances which could be harmful when taken in large quantities. It is best to do your own experimentation in small steps. We are not prescribing or even recommending. We are recording and relating nature's cures as used by the Hawaiians and other Polynesians—nature's offering to all of us.

4

Other Medical Secrets of the Hawaiians and Polynesians

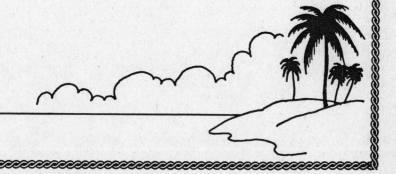

Foods and herbs can be nature's best medicines. Some have been so successful that they still survive today among the Hawaiians and Polynesians. In the following chapters, we will reveal the foods that keep you youthful and well, but in this chapter are the old-time remedies for such conditions as:

LOW ENERGY	*DURING PREGNANCY*
SINUS	*EASING DELIVERY*
SORE THROAT	*LIFE EXTENSION*
HANGOVER	*MALE VIRILITY*
OPEN SORES	*GENERAL DEBILITY*
BABY'S RASHES	*INFECTIONS*
SORE EYES	*PAIN*
KIDNEY PROBLEMS	*TENSION*
POSTNATAL RECOVERY	*CONGESTION*
COMMON COLD	*FEVER*
ULCERS	*EARACHE*
WORMS	*HEMORRHOIDS*
SYSTEMS IMBALANCE	*SKIN PROBLEMS*
ABORTION	*URINARY*
CONCEPTION	*BRONCHITIS*
NAUSEA	*ASTHMA*

DYSENTERY	*COLD SORES*
CONSTIPATION	*DIABETES*
SEASICKNESS	*GOUT*
WARTS	*HEART PROBLEMS*
CORNS	*INSECT REPELLENT*
HEADACHE	*BACKACHE*
LABOR PAINS	*DRY BREASTS*
INDIGESTION	*RHEUMATISM*
TOOTHACHE	*HALITOSIS*
POOR CIRCULATION	*CANKER SORES*
CANCER	

The biggest crop exported by Hawai'i happens to be one of the greatest hazards to health today. Little wonder that Hawaiians want to get rid of their sugar. It is the principal cause of America's obesity problem and all of the ailments attendant on excess weight.*

But the Hawaiians did use sugar cane to improve their health. Here is their secret.

They used the juice of the raw cane. The juice was drained from pounded cane stalks, strained and either boiled first or drunk fresh.

LOW ENERGY. One old Hawaiian gentleman told us that his father drank this sugar cane juice as a tonic every morning. It not only gave his father quick energy to start the day's work, but it was also a tonic for any member of the family who felt weak or debilitated. It acted as quickly as a modern "shot in the arm."

Sugar cane is not native to Hawai'i. It was brought here by the Polynesian settlers who later became the Hawaiian people. Some of the cane was eaten on the trip—the stalks chewed and the juice swallowed—to keep the travelers hardy during the rugged voyage. The rest was planted on arrival.

There were different types of cane then. The white cane, called *kokea,* was reserved for the high-ranking chiefs *(ali'i)* and their families. Plots where these cream-colored stalks, streaked with pale green, were grown were marked *"kapu"* (forbidden to commoners).

---

*For further information on sugar as a weight factor, see *Petrie's Miracle-3 Diet for Guaranteed Weight Loss,* Petrie with Stone, Parker Publishing Company.

Other kinds of cane were available to the common people, and these evolved into the variety that is prevalent in Hawai'i today.

Recently, the practice of "juicing" cane was revived. The result is a product called Sugar Canestrap, a natural and nutritious sweetener that bears none of the death-dealing dangers of refined sugar. It is gradually being introduced into health food stores across the country, but if it's not available yet in your area, you may write for more information to Sugar Cane Products, Inc., 3003 Nimitz Highway, Honolulu, Hawaii 96819.

This "honey of the tall grass" is excellent for a topping on breads, cereals and ice cream, or in coffee and tea. It is pure tropical energy.

It takes a pound of *ko,* the Hawaiian name for sugar cane, to make one ounce of this thick syrup brewed from the juice. We hear that it is also being exported from Puerto Rico, but when you get it from Honolulu, you are enjoying Hawai'i's sweetest *aloha.*

SWEETS THAT ARE GOOD FOR YOU

The closer you get to the raw cane juice, the better the sugar will be for you. Perhaps we should say, "the less harmful it will be for you," because it is only the raw cane juice itself that can be called a desirable tonic.

Raw sugar is frequently available in supermarkets, especially on the West Coast where sugar refining takes place. Raw sugar is better than refined white sugar. Even brown sugar is better than white sugar, although it is really white sugar with some of the molasses—a product of the refining process—put back into it.

Many Hawaiians realize that even honey is better for them than sugar, and local blossoms that light up the islands all year round provide a natural source of this sweetener. However, we have no evidence that Hawai'i's honey is any better for you than honey derived from mainland bee hives.

SINUS; SORE THROAT. Another sweet, brought to the islands by the Chinese, is licorice. Although originally a perennial European plant of the pea family, licorice *(Glycyrrhiza glabra)* became respected in China for its medicinal value, and Hawaiians owe its presence to the original Chinese who settled here. Their descendants still use it for relieving sinus problems and also for soothing sore throats.

Be careful when buying licorice, though. Make sure it is the real thing. Too many of the black candy sticks sold in American stores are synthetic. And be wary of eating too much of even the natural licorice. It can cause high blood pressure.

A California businessman, who once traveled the world designing shopping centers, became so impressed with the licorice he found in other countries that he opened a licorice emporium that has gained the reputation for being the "licorice headquarters" of the United States. George Mazurik's Licorice Shop is in Manhattan Beach, California.

REMARKABLE CHINESE AND FILIPINO DISCOVERIES STILL PRACTICED IN HAWAI'I

Although the Polynesians of the South Pacific are believed to have been the first settlers of the Hawaiian Island chain, there is evidence, in the form of petroglyphs carved on lava rock near the sea, that ancient voyagers from China, possibly via the Philippines, visited these islands long before the Polynesians.

Certainly the Chinese and Philippine people were among the first to add their cultures to today's exotic mixture.

Each culture has contributed its own health secrets, still practiced despite intermarriages.

HANGOVER. Have you had too much beer? Do what your Filipino neighbors advise: Make a gruel of chopped potatoes and onions. Eat a liberal portion and say, "goodbye, hangover."

OPEN SORES. If you have access to guava trees, the tips of the leaves, boiled and mashed into a poultice and placed on open sores, will cause them to heal amazingly fast.

BABY'S RASHES. Certainly you have access to mother's milk. Despite the popularity of modern formula methods, breastfeeding is still done—and preferred by many in Hawai'i. Mother's milk, rubbed into baby's rashes, results in quick relief.

SORE EYES. And if mother's eyes are sore—or those of anybody else in the neighborhood—a few drops of her milk will provide soothing help.

KIDNEY PROBLEMS. The Philippine people add another health use to the long list of properties of the ubiquitous coconut. Kidney trouble, they say, responds to daily quaffs of the coconut water. We heard about some impressive results when coconut water was imbibed daily. This means that you need to buy the whole inside of the husked coconut, sometimes available in supermarkets but more frequently found in the specialty grocery stores. Shake the coconut first to make sure that the water is still in it.

Food is nature's best medicine. That precept is ascribed to by many cultures, starting right from childbirth.

POSTNATAL RECOVERY. Jackie L., a Caucasian, married a Chinese man. Right after the birth of her first child, her mother-in-law fixed her a concoction and insisted that she eat some every day.

"What is it, Mom?"

"Eat it. It's good for you."

Jackie's body restored itself quickly. She had no postpartum discomforts and none of the depression that is usually so common after delivery. She continued eating her daily portions of this mysterious concoction for 30 days, and felt marvelous.

Later, she found out the ingredients: pig's feet, slices of ginger and eggs, simply cooked together.

Jackie's mother-in-law also used the guava tree, which grows only in southern and western states. She used the leaf buds to make a tea. As soon as Jackie returned from the hospital with her baby, her mother-in-law gave her some of the tea to bathe her sexual parts and some to drink. Postpartum soreness disappeared rapidly and she felt that she was being cleansed internally by the tea she drank.

HEALING PROPERTIES OF THE "STINKING ROSE"

Marco Polo brought spaghetti back from China to Italy, but one wonders whether he could have exchanged garlic for it. The Chinese have a high regard for the healing qualities of the "stinking rose."

Known more scientifically as *allium satirum,* this first cousin to the lily was popularized in Hawai'i largely by the Chinese people who came here. But you can get "yes" votes for the therapeutic value of garlic from many cultures.

A Moslem legend says that garlic sprang from the ground at the left foot of Satan when he walked in the Garden of Eden, and onions sprang up at his right foot.

Persians, as early as the tenth century, believed that garlic was an antidote for deadly poisons and that it repelled snakes. It is known today that the crude extract of garlic kills mosquitoes and cures worms, the latter being the reason why it is put in dog food, besides the fact that dogs have an instinctive liking for it.

The Persians also claimed for garlic its ability to stop toothache "if you bruise it and lay it upon the tooth," and to grow hair.

Russian folk medicine prescribed garlic in vodka for arteriosclerosis and as an old age tonic.

In ancient Egypt, garlic was worshipped and 15 pounds of it would buy a slave.

COMMON COLD. Today, the Chinese in Hawai'i recommend garlic as a cure for the common cold. They make a soup of garlic, ginger and watercress, adding the usual vegetable or meat soup stock and simmering the mixture until all the ingredients are soft. The Chinese have another popular cure for colds. They salt whole lemons, using Hawaiian or kosher-type salt. They store these salted lemons in a jar, keeping the jar in sunlight or a warm place for several months, the longer the better. Then, when a cold strikes, they break a salted lemon into a cup, add hot water and drink. Many Chinese homes in Honolulu store salted lemons in this way, and the local herbalists always have them on hand.

ULCERS. Chinese eat raw garlic as a cure for ulcers. They break off a bud from the cluster, remove the outer skin, chew the bud until all the juice has been extracted and then swallow the rest.

Garlic is, of course, available in all food stores. But if you do not like the taste of garlic, you can buy garlic oil in capsule form at most health food stores and some drug stores.

WORMS. Garlic is still highly recommended as a worm-killer. In the old days, before the modern capsule was invented, children and others who did not like the taste of garlic were instructed to walk on it. Small cloves of garlic were placed in each shoe. As the garlic was crushed by walking, its worm-killing oil entered the skin and was carried by the blood into the intestines where the worms reside. Garlic oil has a high penetrating ability. You can prove this to yourself by rubbing some garlic into your skin. In ten minutes have somebody smell your breath: "Hey, you've been eating garlic!"

KEEPING THE BODY IN BALANCE

The general philosophy of ancient Hawaiian medicine concerned itself with the control of body fluids such as the blood, lymph and bile. These fluids are known as body humors. Bad humors in balance with good humors make for body health, all of which is quite similar to the Chinese beliefs.

SYSTEMS IMBALANCE. Medicinal plants and herbs keep the physiological systems clear and purged of roadblocks to good health. There are some ten plants or plant parts that have been used to keep the body in balance. Of these, two are commonly available and three are harder to come by.

Watercress and hibiscus are available to you. Watercress is an excellent salad ingredient and it makes a tasty soup condiment or vegetable. (See recipes in Chapter 11.)

The hibiscus flower, also known in its northern form as the rose of Sharon, is available as an herb tea. Hawaiians feed the hibiscus blossom petals to babies. And the Hawaiian babies are among the healthiest in the world.

Three other plants used in systems balancing, but probably not easily available to you, are:

Hawaiian Name	Botanical Name	Common Name
Koali'awa	Ipomoea insularis	Native morning glory
Koali-pehu	Ipomoea dissecta	Moon flower
Hapu'u	Heart of young shoots	Tree fern

Just a reminder: Some species of mainland morning glory are poisonous.

MORE CHILDBEARING TIPS FROM THE PACIFIC

The Hawaiian, Chinese and Filipino cultures are rich in beliefs and practices for the childbearing period.

We have already mentioned licorice in this chapter. It was used by women as an aphrodisiac, to give them more sexual desire. And in a moment we will be telling you about *ginseng*—the male aphrodisiac.

Rural Hawaiian women believed in the contraceptive power of certain herb teas that grew locally. They could also induce abortion through the use of extracts of herbs found locally.

ABORTION. Two food items purported to induce abortion and used by both Hawaiian and Philippine young women are the skin of the pomegranate fruit boiled and then dried, and the horseradish root boiled until tender.

CONCEPTION. On the other hand, to aid in conception, Philippine women make a drink consisting of meal ground from pear skin, green grass and tree bark.

NAUSEA. If there was nausea in the early days of pregnancy, ginger tea was said to be the answer. Peppermint tea was also used, but we believe that this was introduced later by Westerners.

DURING PREGNANCY. Hawaiians advised their pregnant women against eating any spicy foods: "It can get into the baby's eyes." They also advised against salty foods and, for the duration, one of their favorite foods—raw fish—was also eliminated.

EASING DELIVERY. Both Hawaiians and Filipinos believed, and still do, that raw eggs taken before the baby was expected would ease the whole process of delivery.

POSTNATAL RECOVERY. We have already mentioned the pig's feet cooked with ginger and eggs as a postnatal tonic. Another favorite may not come as a surprise. It is chicken soup, which has been recently confirmed as having therapeutic value by members of the medical profession. Chicken soup has been used by the Hawaiians for centuries to build strength during recovery from childbirth or illness.

A SEX-BUILDING, LIFE-EXTENDING ROOT

Take a walk along the streets of Honolulu's Chinatown and in the window of store after store, you will see a root displayed that looks remarkably like the figure of a man. It is called *ginseng.*

Ginseng is the root of a plant that used to grow in China. It has red berries in the fall. After several years of growth, the root begins to grow branches. Quite commonly, these branches stick out sideways at the top near the neck, attached to the stalk of the plant, and look like arms. Two branches commonly extend downward at the bottom like legs. And frequently there is a small extension between the legs that is reminiscent of the male sex organ.

Indeed, it is the male organ that is said to benefit from *ginseng*. The reason *ginseng* is no longer found in China is that it was so prized as an aphrodisiac that it was thoroughly harvested and became extinct.

But we have good news for you. For nearly 100 years, *ginseng* has been found in the United States and Canada. Once picked, dried and collected by local dealers, it is usually sent to New York City where Hong Kong merchants compete for it.

Korean *ginseng* is found in most health food stores today. It is well packaged for easy use as tea and is cleverly marketed. But American *ginseng* is much more powerful and highly prized by the Chinese who know their *ginseng*. They are willing to pay several times the price for American *ginseng* than for the Korean variety. In fact, most will turn up their noses at the Korean product if the American *ginseng* is available.

It is becoming more and more scarce but the states in which it grows wild most abundantly are Pennsylvania, Ohio, Virginia, West Virginia, Kentucky and Tennessee.

Ginseng is also cultivated by farmers in the states of Ohio, Wisconsin and Minnesota, as well as in the province of Ontario, Canada.

If you wish to obtain it for free by going on a *ginseng* hunt, check your library for pictures and local literature on its whereabouts. Hide and fur dealers, as well as junkyards, are likely purchasers of *ginseng* locally and can give you information and possibly even sell you a few roots.

Otherwise, it is rushed off to New York City wholesalers and then to Hong Kong.

LIFE EXTENSION. Chinese men, on their death beds, have drunk *ginseng* tea and been able to extend their lives for a few days in order to give them time to straighten out their affairs.

MALE VIRILITY. Others have taken *ginseng* tea or chewed small pieces of the root to continue their virility into old age.

The most common way of preparing *ginseng* tea is to put a small root or piece of a root into a pot with water. Brew it as a tea. After you have drunk the tea, add more water and keep it on the range ready to brew for your next day's cup.

GENERAL DEBILITY. The Chinese place *ginseng* root slices into chicken for flavor and as a general tonic. They will also chew a piece for hours, as we chew gum, and then swallow it.

Sorry, ladies, *ginseng* is not believed to affect the feminine sex as an aphrodisiac. The Chinese divide life energy into two forms, *Yin* and *Yang*—feminine and masculine. The *ginseng* root has masculine life energy. But since there are both energies in each sex, even though one is dominant, a mild tonic benefit can still be experienced by women. We suggest that the Korean *ginseng* in such cases would be adequate, and is easier to use as a tea.

SOME GIFTS OF NATURE WITH SPECIFIC HEALTH BENEFITS

We go to the drugstore for cures and remedies, and we usually pay a fancy price. The Hawaiians and Polynesians used to walk out of their huts and shacks for a few feet and were able to find cures and remedies for the same health problems—free of charge.

INFECTIONS; PAIN. A common weed, plantain, was always within reach. Seeds from this weed were first roasted, then ground with salt and water to form a paste. Placed on boils or infections and left overnight, this paste was a household remedy like iodine. And it was free. The same seeds were also boiled as a tea and taken as a pain killer and for headaches much as we take aspirin. Plantain grows everywhere, including your back yard.

A short walk to the nearest papaya tree brought Hawaiians a quick healing agent for deep cuts. The milky fluid, the sap inside the stalks, was the miracle healer. More will be said in the next chapter about how you can benefit from health secrets of the Hawaiians and Polynesians with the use of papaya and other fruits.

One of the most common, yet revered, of all plants in Hawai'i has been the *ti* plant. Its scientific name is *Cordyline terminalis*. Cuttings for planting are packaged for tourists, so the *ti* plant is growing at least privately all over the United States. It may also be available in your large garden shops.

Ti leaves are considered to be protective. They are used in blessings, such as for a new house where they are placed at each doorway and on all four sides, and in exorcism. In the kitchen, *ti* leaves are used in cooking, as you would use a corn husk, to wrap food.

TENSION; CONGESTION. The *ti* leaves are boiled as tea and the tea is used as a relaxant for nerves and muscles. It is also said to be effective as a decongestant. For this use, the young shoots are boiled together with the leaves in making the tea.

FEVER. When prepared in this way—leaves and young shoots—*ti* tea is also used to lower a dry fever.

EARACHE; SINUS; HEMORRHOIDS. What the Hawaiians call *olena* is the common spice turmeric. However, they used the freshly picked root. They grated it, squeezing the juice through a cloth. The juice was then applied directly to an ear for relief of earache, or used as nose drops for relief of sinus. The turmeric juice was also applied to the anus to relieve hemorrhoids.

You cannot get juice out of the dried turmeric that is sold as spice, so you would have to send away for the root to mail order herbalists, like Erewhon, Inc., 3 East Street, Cambridge, Massachusetts 02141.

OUTSTANDING SAMOAN HEALTH PRACTICES

To the south and west of Hawai'i, about halfway to Australia, lie the islands of Samoa—seven islands of American Samoa and two islands of Western Samoa.

American Samoa is a territory of the United States. Western Samoa, considered by many to be the cradle of the Polynesian race, is an independent country.

It is in Western Samoa that the ancient culture has survived more prevalently and where natural health practices are more in evidence.

These are a healthy, polite and gentle people. No alcohol may be taken into the country, as the Samoan government strictly controls the sale of liquor and beer.

Samoans make a beverage from the root *ava* which is mildly intoxicating in a different manner from alcohol. The drinking of *ava* is usually a ritual reserved for special occasions, and the *ava* bowl is passed around for all to drink from before village fetes and dances.

Here are some of the Samoan health practices which we can borrow, thanks to the availability in the United States of the herbs, trees or plants.

We've already mentioned turmeric. The Samoans have many different uses for it. In fact, turmeric emerges as a major health secret of Hawai'i and Polynesia in its broad applications. Some of these uses do not require the liquid to be squeezed from the root, but merely the application of the turmeric spice externally, and we have known people who have gotten good results from drinking a tea made of the powdered spice.

SKIN PROBLEMS. The external uses of turmeric by Samoans include treatment for skin ulcers, skin rashes and pimples. It is also placed on the navel of a newborn child to speed its healing.

URINARY; BRONCHITIS; ASTHMA. Internally, Samoans use the turmeric juice—and you might try the tea—as a diuretic, and also as an aid to recovery from bronchitis and fever. It is also taken internally in the treatment of asthma.

An important reminder: All herb substances taken as medication should be used in minute quantities at first, in order to ascertain your tolerance. Many of these plants contain substances which in large quantities could be harmful.

DYSENTERY. The banana is a medicine in Samoa when used in a special way. A young Samoan "talking chief" named Imo explained that if you take a green or unripe banana, peel it and then charcoal broil it, you have an excellent treatment for dysentery. Eat one slightly scorched banana, he said, for an end to "the runs."

CONSTIPATION. The opposite results, said Imo, can be obtained from the cream of coconut. This rises to the top of the coconut milk. You can buy frozen coconut milk, defrost it, let it stand in a cool place and use the cream that rises to the top. Cream of coconut is an effective laxative.

Talking Chief Imo was also enthusiastic about a Samoan cure for arthritis:

"Take a coconut, not too old," he said. "Empty out coconut water. You can drink it. It is good. But it is not the cure. Put ocean water in place of the coconut water. Let it stand in the kitchen for three or four weeks. Now, when you pour out the sea water, you will find that the coconut meat is soft like custard. This is the cure for arthritis that we use. Eat this soft coconut meat with a piece of dark bread."

Imo explained that many Samoan families keep these coconuts filled with sea water on hand regularly in case somebody gets an upset stomach from nerves or emotions: "It cures that, too."

OPEN SORES. You can buy coconut oil. Samoans use coconut oil to heal open sores and wounds, while we confine our use of it to the skin as a moisturizer and sunburn deterrent. More will be said about coconuts and bananas in the next chapter.

Citrus fruits, mostly limes and oranges, grow in abundance on Samoa. The limes are used both as a food and a medicine.

NAUSEA. Eating the skinned lime fruit is a common Samoan treatment for nausea.

SORE THROAT. The juice of the lime is gargled to relieve a sore throat.

The juice of the lime is also used on the skin to relieve infections caused by poisonous plants. Since poison ivy and poison sumach do not grow in Samoa or Hawai'i, or at least are not known by that name, we have no way of knowing whether the skin irritation caused by these particular poisonous plants would respond to lime juice. An adventuresome reader might try it on a portion of the rash to test its effectiveness. The lime juice is used undiluted.

SEASICKNESS. Traveling by canoe between their far-flung islands, Samoans needed a way to avoid seasickness. They brought limes aboard with them and, whenever someone sensed that feeling coming on, he would cut a lime and hold half of it up to his nose. All it took to make a good Samoan seaman was a sturdy paddle and a few limes.

CURES FROM OTHER SOUTH PACIFIC ISLANDS

Scores of medicines now prescribed by Western physicians had their origins in natural foods, herbs, seeds and growing substances, and a good fraction of these originated in Hawai'i and Polynesia.

Some of these islands have no modern doctors and the people stay healthy through natural remedies. Unfortunately, the bulk of these remedies are not available in the United States, but we have found a few that are.

WARTS; CORNS. In Tonga, the last remaining Polynesian kingdom with a real live king and royal family, oil from cashew nuts is said to make warts do a disappearing act. Cashew nut oil is also used by the Tongans to remove corns on the feet.

HEADACHE. In Guam, one of the Mariana Islands, coconut oil is mixed with vinegar in equal parts, thoroughly shaken to combine the two liquids, and applied to the forehead to relieve a headache. A Guamanian woman we met swears by this and says she is planning to market this headache cure in the United States. The mixture needs to be rubbed into the forehead skin gently.

In Fiji, where missionaries used to be invited for dinner only to discover that they were the main course, the people are healthy and vigorous. This is not due to cannibalism, which has long since been stopped, but to the fresh air, fresh fish and fresh fruits and vegetables in abundance. Even malaria, so common in the tropics, is unknown in Fiji.

LABOR PAINS. Labor pains are a fact of life even among a healthy people. To relieve the pains of childbirth, Fijian women drink the juice of hibiscus flowers mixed with lemon juice.

DYSENTERY. We mentioned the *ti* leaves of Hawai'i earlier in this chapter. In Tahiti, an island famous for its special brand of rapid, hip-gyrating hula dance, *ti* leaves are squeezed and the resulting juice mixed with the water of green or unripe coconut as a cure for diarrhea or dysentery. Drink a 5-ounce glassful four times a day.

THE CURATIVE PROPERTIES CLAIMED FOR GINGER

We have mentioned ginger as used in connection with some remedies. The ginger root, obtainable in most supermarkets, was a veritable Hawaiian drugstore.

Known here as *'awapuhi kuahiwi,* and officially as *Zingiber zerumbet,* ginger is a succulent plant with long oval leaves that grow around the stem, enveloping it. Its flowers are yellow, white or red—each from a different type of ginger plant—and quite fragrant.

Plant a ginger root and you may be able to grow your own ginger plant.

Ancient Hawaiians used the juice of the ginger flower as a hair dressing. However, it is the root from which they derived the most benefits.

INDIGESTION. Using a piece of ginger root the size of a small finger, Hawaiians boiled it to extract the essence, let it simmer a few minutes and then drank a cupful before meals to head off chronic indigestion and stomach distress.

TOOTHACHE. For toothache, they cut off a piece of the root and cooked it by rolling it over the red coals of the fire. (You can use a frying pan.) Then they shaped it to fit the hollow of the aching tooth. Biting down on it fixes it in place; then loosen your jaw and let the saliva flow. Usually one application, leaving the piece of root on the tooth for a while, was all that was needed, but you can repeat if necessary.

HEADACHE. The juice of ginger roots, obtained by pounding the root with salt—again, it is better to use kosher salt than the common variety—provided a quick remedy for headaches. Merely rub the salted juice over the pained areas of the head.

The many other remedial uses of the ginger root by the Hawaiians included correcting white blotches on the skin, ringworm, itch, sprains and bruises, and in massage. However, these uses required mixing ginger root with other Hawaiian herbs and plants that are not available elsewhere, and some of which are no longer available even in Hawai'i.

REMEDIES OF UNKNOWN PACIFIC ORIGIN STILL IN USE

Hawai'i's position in the Pacific area has made it the meeting place of many cultures, from Russia and Korea to the north, to New Zealand and Australia to the south.

Its people include combinations of many races and cultures, who have brought with them the successful remedies of their forefathers, often untraceable to their actual place of origin.

Here is a flurry of Hawaiian and Polynesian health practices that have survived for hundreds of years of use, and have been handed down from generation to generation.

POOR CIRCULATION. Boil common *seaweed* in water to extract the iodine and other minerals. Then apply to arms or legs.

CONSTIPATION. Eat a copious amount of fresh *raspberries*. If frozen berries are used, rinse off the sugar water. Another effective remedy is to mix *arrowroot powder* in warm water and drink.

CANCER. Eat *papaya seeds* several times a day for cancer in its early stages.

COLD SORES. Vinegar is applied directly to the cold sore, three or four times daily.

SORE THROAT. Squeeze the juice from a raw *sweet potato,* mix with warm water and gargle.

DIABETES. Drink *coconut water* daily and go on a vegetable diet.

GOUT. Make a *parsley soup*. Drink daily, accompanied by a diet of largely green vegetables. Or, make a *watercress soup*. Drink daily and maintain a vegetarian diet.

HEART PROBLEMS. Drink the juice of *watercress* or eat copious amounts of fresh watercress.

INSECT REPELLENT. Rub the rind of *lemon* on the skin where exposed.

KIDNEY PROBLEMS. Drink *lemon grass* tea, three times daily. Or, make a tea from *rose petals,* and drink several times daily. This appears to be of Maori (New Zealand) origin.

BACKACHE. Wet the leaves from a *geranium* plant and place as a poultice on the aching area.

DRY BREASTS. Chop and cook *papaya* fruit (no seeds) in one quart of water. Add a piece of pork. Mother eats both the papaya gravy and the pork.

RHEUMATISM. Pound *chili pepper* seeds with sea salt (available at health food stores). Rub the mixture into afflicted parts.

OCEAN WATER AS A HEALTH REMEDY

Surrounded by the salt water of the Pacific Ocean, people of these islands found many healthful uses for that ocean water, which we on the continents have long forgotten, if indeed we ever knew them.

COMMON COLD. Sea water is helpful for the common cold. It is a good gargle for relieving a sore throat. When cupped in your hand and sniffed up into your nostrils, it also relieves a "stuffed-up" nose.

HALITOSIS. Used as a gargle by Hawaiians, sea water was said to sweeten bad breath.

INDIGESTION. As a stomach and colon cleanser, salt water was used as both a vomiting inducer and an enema, depending on which area needed cleansing.

CANKER SORES. Gargling with hot sea water is the way in which Japanese pineapple and sugar cane workers get rid of canker sores and irritated gums.

Salt was extracted by the Hawaiians from sea water in a special way that left all of the minerals intact, as opposed to the salt refining processes we use for common table salt, which is derived not from the sea but from mineral salt mines that are largely sodium chloride.

When salt is extracted from the ocean, it contains many minerals that supply bodily needs. Sea salt may be obtained from health food stores and this sea salt is far superior to common mined salt. However, the Hawaiians are still producing sea salt in the old way, especially on the island of Kaua'i where large rock tubs capture sea water at high tide. This water is evaporated by the sun, leaving the salt sediment to be scraped out.

Take home some of this salt if you visit Hawai'i, and use it with the healing remedies that call for salt described earlier in this chapter.

In the next chapter, we will discuss some of the foods that keep Hawaiians healthy and which are probably brimming with Hawaiian sunshine right now in your supermarket, ignored and overlooked by most shoppers.

5

Life-Giving Island
Fruits and Nuts
Available Everywhere

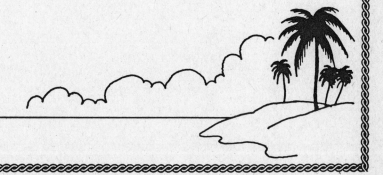

Here are fruits that heal and fruits that "healthify." Here, too, are other tree products—nuts—that provide body building nutrients in concentrated form. After reading this chapter, your menus will change as you add these fruits and nuts for increased vitality. The specific disorders and deficiencies for which these remedies are used by island people include:

HARDENING OF ARTERIES	CONSTIPATION
APPETITE	IMPOTENCY
THROMBOSIS	KIDNEY AILMENTS
ARTHRITIS	FEVER
RHEUMATOID ARTHRITIS	COMMON COLD
MALNUTRITION	STOMACH GAS
ULCERS	LOOSE BOWELS
INTESTINAL INFLAMMATION	TEETH AND GUMS

And the specific health reinforcing qualities include:

VITAMIN A	ALL-PURPOSE
RIBOFLAVIN	LOW-CALORIE
NIACIN	VITAMIN C
FIBER	LIFE ENERGY
POTASSIUM	MEAT TENDERIZER
EASE OF DIGESTION	PAIN RELIEVER
ANTISEPTIC	NERVE TONIC

SLEEP INDUCER   *SKIN MOISTURIZER*
STRENGTH   *HAIR CONDITIONER*
LONGEVITY   *MASSAGE*
BODY BUILDING   *SUNTAN*
ROUGHAGE   *SUPER NUTRITION*
IRON   *VITALITY*
PHOSPHORUS   *FUNGICIDE*

Pacific island people have a high life expectancy.

This means a low incidence of illness.

In this chapter we shift from the negative to the positive—from ways
to use food as medicine to ways to use food to maintain a young, energetic and healthy body.

Ten years ago this chapter could not have been written. Ten years
ago you would have had to come to Hawai'i to gain the benefits that
Hawaiians enjoy. But now, thanks to advances in the transportation of
food, fresh Hawaiian and Polynesian fruit is being flown "fresh from the
tree" to all the major markets of the United States.

You have quite likely been passing up many of these fruits because
they are unfamiliar to you, and instead you have been buying apples,
pears, peaches, grapes and other familiar fruits in season. Nothing we may
say in this chapter is intended to deter you from these fruits. If anything,
the chief lesson taught by the islanders is that we should all eat more fruit
than we do.

"An apple a day keeps the doctor away" is still a trustworthy adage.
Apples are great for you. So are other fruits, melons and berries. They are
much better desserts than pies, cakes, ice cream, tarts and puddings.
"Better" means they cause less illness and bring a higher resistance to
infectious diseases, greater vigor and longer life.

Hawaiian and Polynesian fruits have special qualities. Come to
Hawai'i, in this chapter. Savor the fruits of Paradise and let them reveal
their health secrets to you.

THE "FRUIT OF PARADISE"

Have you eaten a *Musa paradisiaca* recently? That is the technical
name for the banana. In Hawai'i it is called "*maia*" and legend has it here
that the banana, not the apple, was the fruit of the tree of the knowledge

of good and evil—the tempting treat offered to Adam by Eve—thus adding validity to the scientific name *paradisiaca*.

We have our bread and potatoes. The Hawaiians have their bananas. If they would trade their bananas for our bread, they would be making a bad deal, especially if it was the usual white bread that most of us eat.

Bananas, as rich and creamy as they taste, are actually an excellent slimming food. They are filling, yet practically free of fat and moderate in calories. An average 7-inch banana contains only about 120 calories. You would do well in terms of nutrients and calories to trade two slices of bread for a banana.

There are many types of bananas. The most common variety in the United States mainland markets is labeled "Chiquita." It is a product of the United Fruit Company and is obtained largely from Central and South America.

In Hawai'i, "Chiquita" bananas lie side by side in fruit departments with local Hawaiian varieties. Personally, we always buy the Hawaiian variety because it has been off the tree for less time. But so many mainlanders now live on these islands that there are not enough local bananas to go around. Fortunately, the mainlanders prefer the size and shape they became accustomed to in Oshkosh or Jersey City, and so we all have the bananas we like best.

Although there are slight variations in mineral and vitamin content, any banana you buy is good for you. "Chiquita" is usually the Bluefield variety. We will talk about these because the Hawaiian varieties seldom leave these shores. Even if you see the Hawaiian-associated name "Dole" on bananas, they are quite likely grown in some other part of the world and are still the Bluefield variety, although we have some Bluefields growing here, too.

VITAMIN A; RIBOFLAVIN; NIACIN. Bananas are composed of carbohydrates, as are all fruits. The eating varieties contain only about 1 percent protein and 1/10 percent fat. They are high in vitamin A, containing about 200 International Units. They are not a good source of vitamin C, containing less than 10 milligrams, but they are a relatively good source for riboflavin (about 50 micrograms), and for niacin (nearly 1 microgram).

FIBER; POTASSIUM. Bananas are high in fiber and potassium. There is a hidden value, too, in bananas that is not measurable in milligrams or micrograms.

EASE OF DIGESTION. Most fruits require digestive effort by the body. Some "take" almost as much as they "give." Not so with bananas. They are about the easiest fruit to digest. They are "givers."

That is why bananas are a popular infant food. They should be ripe. Unripe bananas may cause digestive problems even with adults. However, when the green banana turns yellow and the yellow becomes flecked with brown spots, the fruit's carbohydrate is becoming transformed into sugar, much like what happens during the digestive process. So you might say that a ripe banana is already partially digested.

That is why your body gains more than it has to give and you wind up with a plus in non-fattening nourishment. Furthermore, bananas are non-acidic and in fact have an alkaline reaction.

ANTISEPTIC. Bananas are kept germ-free for you by nature. The skin of bananas is known as "nature's bacteria-proof wrapper." For centuries people who live in the tropics have been pounding banana peels into a pulp and using it as a poultice on infections and cuts. Today science agrees that the skins of ripe bananas contain a strong antibiotic that is effective against both pathogenic bacteria and disease-causing fungi.

Bananas are available all year round with the hottest months slowing down production slightly and the cooler months accelerating it.

Put them on every shopping list, both the eating kind and the cooking varieties. The latter are not common in the U. S. mainland markets, but you can cook unripe, green bananas by boiling them in their skins for a half-hour. Then peel, slice and top with cream.

Plantain is a tropical fruit that resembles a banana. It is always cooked, because it is not very palatable when eaten raw. If the bananas you buy look different, perhaps longer and thicker, inquire to make sure whether they are bananas or plantain.

Plantain (and unripe or green bananas) can be boiled, fried, baked and broiled. They go well with meats and casseroles, as a vegetable and as a dessert.

ALL-PURPOSE. Eating bananas have a variety of uses besides peeling back the skin and biting off a luscious mouthful. Slice them on cereals, place them in salads or mash them with peanut butter for a sandwich. And when they get overripe, how about banana bread?

Eat a banana today. As you do, imagine that you have picked it off a large stalk of bananas that you cut from a tree a few days ago and placed outside your back door to ripen. Think of its yellow skin as the glorious sunshine of the tropics. Taste its creamy fruit, knowing that it is the fruit of Paradise!

THE TENDERIZER FRUIT

There is a fruit that healthy Hawaiians enjoy equally well for breakfast, lunch or dinner. For years travelers to Hawai'i carried home this fruit which, like the banana, is also green when unripe and bright yellow when fully ripe. But now papaya is famous.

It is flown by jet to the other 49 states and is becoming a more and more familiar sight in supermarkets.

DIGESTIVE AID. Even before papaya became known to housewives, they were using meat tenderizers which depend on the enzyme, papain, that is found in papaya. Papain is a protein-splitting enzyme that not only makes steak more tender and palatable, but helps the digestive system to accomplish its work.

Just as the banana is easy to digest, so is the papaya practically a self-digester.

LOW-CALORIE. Furthermore, a serving of half of an average-sized papaya, a serving that weighs approximately 7 ounces of edible fruit, contains only 80 calories, which, as dieters will note, make it the lowest calorie fruit next to the grapefruit.

VITAMIN A; VITAMIN C; POTASSIUM. In addition, papaya is brimming with vitamin A (3500 units) and vitamin C (112 milligrams). It is high in potassium, containing over 400 milligrams of this essential mineral.

Just about everyone who owns a home with a piece of land in Hawai'i grows papaya. The tree, which is really not a tree but a tall hollow-stemmed plant that can reach a height of 25 to 30 feet, produces fruit within a year of planting from a seed. It is successfully grown in warmer states and has a high degree of recovery from cold or injury. If the "tree" is toppled by a high wind, for instance, the main stem immediately puts out a number of branches.

LIFE ENERGY. This is indicative of the immeasurable life energy in the papaya fruit. Chemical analysts and vitamin counters can "do their thing" but they will never be able to tag their nomenclature on the real life-supporting essence of papaya.

In the previous chapter we told you how the seeds are used for certain cures. Actually, the seeds are not very palatable, so they are spooned away after cutting the fruit into halves.

A ripe papaya spoons out easily and the riper it is the easier it is to eat all the way down to the skin, which is not edible.

If it tastes a bit flat to you, you can add a wedge of lemon or lime to liven it up. Papaya makes a good breakfast fruit. It does more than its share as an ingredient for a luncheon fruit salad. And it makes a healthful dinner dessert.

At the market, do not squeeze the fruit to see if it is soft, for papaya bruises easily. Judge by the color as you would with a banana: bright yellow for immediate use, green with yellow areas for tomorrow or the next day, and totally green for the end of the week.

It is a versatile food. It can be used alone or with other fruits to make a blender drink. It can be roasted with meat and fowl. Ham or seafood salads can be served in papaya halves. It can be used in pancake batter and bread dough. See the recipes in Chapter 11.

MEAT TENDERIZER; PAIN RELIEVER. We frequently rub papaya pulp onto steak and let it stand for a while before broiling. It tenderizes and adds flavor as the enzyme papain goes to work. This enzyme also makes papaya a good first aid measure in drawing pain from insect or jellyfish stings.

If you have walked past the papaya at your market and have never tried it, buy one and taste it. Its taste might be described as reminiscent of a Crenshaw melon with a peach flavor.

Savor its rich tropical sweetness and then regularly give yourself this treat of island vitality.

THE FRUIT WITHOUT A TREE

Fruit, generally speaking, is good for you.

Certain Pacific island fruits are excellent for you.

Every so often, scientists make a discovery about why a certain food is beneficial. Such a discovery has recently been made about the next fruit that we are going to discuss—a fruit that does a Herculean job in boosting health levels in Hawai'i.

That fruit is the pineapple.

No, pineapples do not grow on trees. Tour directors like to joke with visitors about the pineapple tree. Pineapples grow on a low cactus-like plant which averages about 2 feet in height while bearing fruit. The pineapple is called a multiple fruit because it is actually a collection of fruits around a solid core.

Most people are familiar with pineapple slices that come in cans but are not familiar with the fruit itself, which looks something like a large pine cone. The average fruits weighs 5 pounds, but can be as large as 8 pounds. The pineapple is mottled green and brown when picked and as it continues to ripen it becomes more yellow or chocolate brown.

The discovery that scientists are now researching to confirm is that pineapple contains an enzyme called bromelain which is helpful in treating cardiovascular diseases.

HARDENING OF ARTERIES. Hardening of the arteries is one of the killing aspects of aging. Bromelain may be the answer. Initial studies indicate that it is an artery cleanser and might very well clear arteries of the sludge which hardens them and blocks smaller capillaries, thus contributing to senility.

As research continues, bromelain is being made available to the public in concentrated form. One such product is "Anavit" which is innocently described on its label as "a dietary supplement of vitamin C with the natural enzyme system of pineapple." Ingredients are described as "derived from natural sources—no sucrose or artificial sweetener, coloring, flavoring or preservatives added." They are listed as dried whey, 75 milligrams of Hawaiian bromelain with 90 Geletin Digestion Units per tablet, 15 milligrams of vitamin C and corn protein.

Geletin Digestion Units are a measure of the enzyme strength of the bromelain.

The pineapple enzyme bromelain is a highly sensitive biological material. It is easily damaged during processing into tablets. It took some ten years of research and experience by its makers, Chemical Consultants International, Inc.,* to finally produce a highly active yet stable form.

Reports have filtered in from physicians in various parts of the United States who have used bromelain for patients and have found it to be ineffective. These reports, when investigated, usually reveal that the

---

*P.O. Box 88041, Honolulu, Hawaii 96815.

brand of bromelain used was far less active or strong than what the label stated.

We are fortunate in Hawai'i to have the brand name Anavit because it is made entirely in Hawai'i where more people know more about pineapple and pineapple enzymes than anywhere else in the world.

Anavit with the green label, the strength of which was described above, has been joined by Anavit-F3, a stronger version. While regular green label Anavit requires three to nine tablets per day before or during meals, yellow label Anavit-F3 requires only one to four tablets per day. Once opened, Anavit needs to be refrigerated.

ANANAS ARE NOT BANANAS

Most of the world knows pineapple as *ananas*. It grows in the Caribbean, the Philippines and southeast Asia. Its health properties have been known for centuries. Here is an excerpt from *History of the Carribby Islands*, by Charles de Rochfort, published in France in 1658:

> The Ananas or Pine-Apple is accounted the most deli-
> cious fruit, not only of these islands, but of all America. It is so
> delightful to the eye, and so sweet a scent, that Nature may be
> said to be extremely prodigal of what was most rare and pre-
> cious in her Treasury to this Plant . . .
> APPETITE. In Physick the virtues of it are there–the juice
> does admirably recreate and exhilarate the Spirits and comfort
> the Heart; it also fortifies the stomach . . . and causeth Appe-
> tite. It gives present ease to such as are troubled with the
> Stone, or stoppage of Urine. Nay, it destroys the force of
> poison. If the fruit be not procurable, the root will do the same
> effect.

It is in fact the stalk and other portions of the plant that are the present sources of bromelain for concentrated use, the fruit being too good to use for this purpose and the wonder enzyme being just as available, if not more so, from the stalk as from the fruit.

If you would like to go behind the scenes of current medical research on bromelain—and that is the only way to get to the core of the exciting medical discoveries being made, as it will not be publicized until all government regulations and requirements have been met—you must read technical papers and reports in medical journals.

Let us give you a peek into the *Hiroshima Journal of Medical Sciences*. In the September 1975 issue of this Japanese publication, there appeared an article written by two American researchers, Steven J. Taussig, Ph.D., of Honolulu, and Allen Chinen, B.S., of Stanford University in Palo Alto, California, and two Japanese medical doctors, M. Mitsu Yokoyama and Yukio Nishimoto. Here are some excerpts:

> *THROMBOSIS. Bromelain—a long overlooked compound—promises an impressive number of medical uses. Particularly in inflammation, edema, burn and recently thrombosis therapy. Bromelain is being extensively tested today. Ironically, although bromelain is well-known in Japan and South America, and is almost a household word in Europe, relatively few physicians in the U. S. know of it.*
>
> *ARTHRITIS. Bromelain is effective in the treatment of trauma, edema and inflammation. Generally administered orally, bromelain is useful in general and oral surgery. It is also used alone or as an adjunct therapy in arthritis, cellulitis, thrombophlebitis, and pulmonary edema.*

RHEUMATOID ARTHRITIS. A physician in Hawai'i told us that he has seen dramatic results when bromelain is used to help rheumatoid arthritis. We have also heard of it being helpful in cancer treatment. Since research is still in its early stages, we predict that the world will be hearing much more about the healing qualities and applications of bromelain, as well as the healthful properties of the pineapple fruit itself.

Unlike both banana and papaya, which tend to start the digestive process in their own ripening, pineapple does not get any sweeter once it is picked, only softer. The sweeter pineapples are those picked in the summer when the days are longer and when the leaves of the plant have had more time to transfer their sugars to the fruit.

It is hard to tell a ripe pineapple in the market by its color. Some people like to pull a leaf from the crown. If it comes off easily, the fruit is believed to be ripe. This is not as dependable a test as snapping with the thumb and finger. A hollow thud is usually made by a not well-matured fruit, but a dull solid sound promises a sounder, juicier fruit.

Don't wait until you finish this book. Buy a fresh pineapple. Don't settle for the canned juice or canned fruit if you can find the whole fruit.

LIFE ENERGY. Slice off the prickly rind. Cut out the hard inner core. And savor the fruit in all its luscious, juicy, natural form, rich in bromelain. You are eating of the fruit of the tree of life. (Pineapple deserves this title, even if it doesn't grow on a tree!)

A FRUIT FOR THE STARVING

MALNUTRITION. There is a fruit that grows wild in Hawai'i, and is available in your supermarket, which is so high in nutrition that it is often recommended to people suffering from malnutrition.

The Aztecs cultivated this fruit in Mexico and called it *"ahaucatl."* When the Spaniards came, they found it easier to call it *"aguacate."* The English further corrupted the sound to "avocado."

Avocados are now sometimes called alligator pears and, in Hawai'i, just pears. Here they are in such abundance that they are frequently fed by farmers to pigs and other livestock. Even dogs and cats will eat the oily fruit, thrive and grow fat.

Fat is the chief ingredient of the avocado. It is one of our few sources of natural oil, and not only does it come in ready-to-eat form but it is also succulent and delicious. Hardly a health food restaurant does not serve guacamole—mashed avocado mixed with chopped garlic, tomato, salt, pepper and lemon juice.

Because of the oil, the avocado is not a weight-loss food. It is high in calories, but also high in vitamins, high in minerals and, therefore, high in healthful nutrition. Vitamins A, B and C are present in significant amounts, as well as calcium, phosphorus and potassium. The B factors include thiamine and riboflavin.

ULCERS. The smooth texture of the avocado fruit has made it an easy food for ulcer sufferers to handle, with few of the digestive problems caused by harsher foods.

INTESTINAL INFLAMMATION; CONSTIPATION. It is also used in Hawai'i by people who have inflammation of the small intestines and colon. Again, its oily quality seems to lubricate its way through the sensitive passages. For this reason, it has been said to be helpful in cases of constipation.

NERVE TONIC; SLEEP INDUCER. It is understandable that a food endowed with such nutritive values as the avocado should be given credit for a multitude of curative powers. We have heard that it has helped in cases of nervousness. One elderly woman of Japanese descent told us that it helped her to fall asleep. The stomach-coating quality of warm milk, known by our forefathers to be a sleep inducer, may have a competitor in the avocado.

IMPOTENCY. More than one person has whispered to us that it is good as a corrective for male impotency.

This could be due to its high mineral content, but then again, there is something strange about the avocado tree's own sex life which might also be a factor: The flower opens, then closes, then opens again. The first time it opens, every flower behaves as if it were a female flower, able to be pollinated but not of itself able to shed pollen. The second time it opens, usually 12 to 24 hours later, it is essentially a male flower, shedding pollen but not in a condition to be pollinated. No other fruit tree is known to behave in this way.

There is no doubt that, as a nutritional food available all year round, the avocado packs a wallop.

YOUR TROPICAL FRUIT BOWL

The healthful radiance of tropical living is now available to everyone, without the need for a plane ticket. Planeloads of tropical fruit are arriving at all major United States markets. Some of these fruits are slow to catch on. But now papaya sales are booming and fresh pineapples are seen as frequently as the canned variety.

Some new fruits—new to the mainland but old friends to island people—are now gaining acceptance as they join the trek north, bringing tropical sunshine to your table even in the dead of the winter.

If you see mangoes, buy them. In Hawai'i they are so profuse that they fall from the trees and rot in the roads faster than they can be collected and enjoyed. The mango fruit is prized wherever mango trees grow. It is considered to be one of the most delicious of all tropical fruits.

Unlike the avocado, which is available at all supermarkets all year round, the mango trees ripen in season only and appear in the markets for only a short time, even in Hawai'i.

So the fruit is made quickly into jams, marmalades, chutneys and breads.

All types of mangoes are excellent sources of vitamin A. Some are good ascorbic acid sources (vitamin C) but this is not dependable.

STRENGTH; KIDNEY AILMENTS. Mangoes come from huge trees and are said to bring to the consumer of the fruit the strength of those trees. More specific health benefits claimed for the mango fruit include help for nephritis, inflammation of the kidneys, and other kidney ailments.

FEVER; COMMON COLD. We have heard of incidents where eating mangoes has helped to reduce fever, but we have no specifics on how many people have been helped, or how often. We have also heard people say that mangoes are good for the common cold. But again, we have no specifics.

Another fruit appearing at supermarkets for brief periods—buy it when you see it—is the kiwi.

LONGEVITY. This exotic sub-tropical fruit comes from New Zealand, the land of the Maoris, who are believed to be closely related to the Hawaiians. In New Zealand, it is regarded as a food that adds to longevity.

VITAMIN C. The kiwi is often called a type of gooseberry. Its interior has the same texture as the inside of the gooseberry. You eat it by cutting it in half and spooning out the deliciously sweet fruit right down to the skin. Super rich in vitamin C, this fruit is flown to the United States from "down under" in the middle of the U. S. winter, bringing with it the cold-resistant qualities of the sunny New Zealand clime. If you would like to know where and when kiwis become available in your area, write to Turners and Growers, Ltd., P.O. Box 56, Auckland, New Zealand.

There are many tropical fruits that contribute to the long life of Hawaiians and Polynesians which you can enjoy only by coming to the islands: guava (you might find them canned), star fruit, pomelo, bread fruit, passion fruit and many others.

But you can find a taste of the tropics in your supermarket: oranges, grapefruit, bananas, papayas, pineapple, avocado and maybe the kiwi and others.

What a delicious and healthful fruit salad!

HAWAI'I'S HEALTH NUTS

People are health-conscious in Hawai'i. The great outdoors is never taken for granted and the availability of fresh, sun-drenched fruits and vegetables is always appreciated. Everyone here is a health nut.

And on every coconut tree there is a health nut.

The coconut is seldom harvested and processed in Hawai'i. Everyone eats them, and grows healthy. But no one wants to spend the time themselves to open them and extract the meat.

So coconuts that are taken from the trees to prevent them from falling on someone's head are tossed into the city dump with one hand and brought in from other parts of the Pacific ready to eat with the other hand.

As recently as ten years ago, we remember the familiar sight of a Hawaiian beach boy shimmying up a palm tree to the top, cutting off a coconut and sliding nimbly down with it. He would then whack it open deftly, make a hole and pass it around for all to enjoy a drink.

If you too are intimidated by the task of opening up the coconut—for even with the stubborn husk off, the inner nut is itself a challenge—then let us show you the lazy way to get at the delicious white meat.

Use an ice pick or a hammer and large nail to pierce three holes at the top of the shell. You may locate one or two "eyes" of the coconut. It is easier to pierce here. Drain off the juice to drink or use for cooking (see recipes in Chapter 11). Heat the coconut in a 375-degree oven for about 20 minutes. The shell will quite likely crack of its own accord. If not, strike it lightly with a hammer, first here and then there until it cracks open.

The food that awaits you is worth the effort.

Actually, the coconut is the fruit of the coconut tree, with one seed inside. When you tear off the fibrous husk, the 4- to 5-inch hard-shelled nut with all the goodies in it, and which you can occasionally buy in your supermarket, is the seed from which another coconut tree would otherwise grow.

Once opened, the white meat on the inside is what most people are familiar with only as the filling for certain types of chocolate candy bars or as the shreds in the coconut icing on a cake. This properly cancels out the healthy uses of the coconut meat. It is sweet enough to eat without negating its nutritive value by adding nutrition-sapping sugar.

The milk and meat of the coconut have been a Hawaiian and Polynesian staple for centuries, just as the stately coconut palms offering beauty, shade and shelter have been an essential part of the South Seas paradise.

However, the liquid you will find in your supermarket coconut is nothing like the liquid of the "drinking" coconut. A "drinking" coconut is one in which you hear no sloshing when you shake it, it is so fully packed. A "drinking" coconut is picked green off the tree and enjoyed on the spot. It is nature's elixir. There is a Hawaiian song that praises the sensation of cool coconut water coursing down a thirsty throat.

THE PALM TREE'S CONTRIBUTION TO HEALTH

Coconut milk is available frozen or in cans in your supermarket. The shredded coconut meat comes dried in paper or plastic bags and can be found in the baking department of every supermarket.

Other coconut products, such as those marketed for ten years now by Noh Foods, include a dehydrated powdered drink to which you merely add water, and Hawaiian Haupia pudding, a delicious easy-to-prepare dessert.

BODY BUILDING. Coconut milk is 27 percent vegetable fat which, like the avocado fat, does not contribute to cholesterol blood levels. Although coconut milk has only 4 percent protein, it is an easily metabolized protein. Hawaiian and Polynesian health uses include giving coconut milk and coconut meat to thin and emaciated people for the building up of body tissues and muscles.

STOMACH GAS; LOOSE BOWELS. There are a number of digestive problems that coconut meat is said to relieve, such as excessive gas in the stomach and cases of inflamed intestines causing loose or bloody evacuations.

ROUGHAGE. Although not a good source for vitamins, the coconut is packed with minerals and is an excellent source of crude fiber, now regarded as important to all diets for the prevention of intestinal diseases.

IRON; PHOSPHORUS. Coconut milk is not a substitute for cow's milk, as it is low in calcium, but it is an excellent source of iron and phosphorus.

A SPECIAL OIL FOR THE BODY

Besides being used by the ancient Hawaiians and Polynesians for food, fire, shelter, utensils and decorations, the coconut provided an oil that they used to beautify their bodies.

Coconut oil is often obtainable in drugstores and pharmacies as a suntan lotion. Unfortunately, it is frequently mixed with other ingredients.

Here is how to extract the oil from the meat of the fresh coconuts you buy in the supermarket produce department. Add boiling water to the grated meat and allow it to sit for one hour. Hand squeeze the milk from the grated meat and cook it over a low heat slowly until the oil rises to the top. Skim it off and strain it.

SKIN MOISTURIZER; HAIR CONDITIONER. Coconut oil is a natural skin moisturizer. The hair, which is really an extension of the skin, also responds well to coconut oil. So it is used successfully as a dry hair conditioner.

MASSAGE. The famous Hawaiian massage, known as *lomi lomi* and which we will discuss later, is usually performed using coconut oil as the skin lubricant.

SUNTAN. The most common use is, of course, as a suntan lotion. Warning: Coconut oil is not a sun screen. The burning rays will get through. However, the oil does help to create an even tan. Be sure to limit your time in the sun with the oil as carefully as you would with no oil.

OTHER HAWAIIAN AND POLYNESIAN NUTS YOUR BODY CAN ENJOY

Nuts are health food.

It is possible to live on only fruits and nuts, and there is a good chance you could live longer that way.

One of the nuts that Hawai'i is most noted for is the macadamia. About 95 percent of the world's supply comes from Hawai'i and practically all of this is grown on the Big Island.

SUPER NUTRITION. These nuts are all but impossible to crack, so the macadamia nuts you buy in glass jars in your supermarket are the de-nutted meats, ready to eat. And they are delicious. They are also super-nutritious. And fattening.

Unfortunately, macadamia nuts are so good and so good for you, there is a big promotion on to increase their sales via chocolate candy, candy brittle and jam. Partaking of macadamia nuts this way is not the Hawaiian way.

If you want to extract the goodness of macadamia nuts for your taste buds as well as your body, stick to the pure meat of the nut, unpolluted with sugar products.

Here is how the macadamia compares to the peanut, another good food in essential nutrients.

	6 peanuts	Equivalent macadamia
Carbohydrate	85	105
Protein	4.3	1.4
Calcium	8 mg	5 mg
Phosphorus	—	62 mg
Iron	.03	.5
Riboflavin	.018	.21
Niacin	.2	2.8
Fat	11.7	7

Another nut that is popular in Polynesia is the cashew. You are probably quite familiar with this nut. It is grown abundantly in Samoa where it was introduced by people from India and known as the "Indian apple."

TEETH AND GUMS. Children in Samoa love to eat cashew nuts. It is probably an intuitive attraction, because cashews have been reported to be good for teeth and gums.

BODY BUILDING; VITALITY. Cashew nuts also have a reputation for being good body builders, especially in cases of malnutrition or emaciation. Cashew nut butter is easily digested and helps build vitality.

Here in Hawai'i we have the privilege of eating freshly picked lichee nuts. This Chinese delicacy comes to you canned. As delicious as it is canned, it is like "food for the gods" when you get it fresh.

We also have the kukui nut which you see worn as necklaces or leis by men and women alike. There was a time when kukui nut oil was exported by Hawaiians to Alaska, which was then occupied by the Russians. This oil makes a good burning oil for night illumination.

FUNGICIDE. However, the nut itself when burned into charcoal was used against skin diseases caused by fungus.

There are other foods which, like these, are not available except on these islands. But here in this chapter, you have the best of Hawaiian and Polynesian fruits and nuts, which are available to you and which deserve a more prominent place in your menu for healthful living.

6

Other Foods Hawaiians and Polynesians Eat to Stay Young

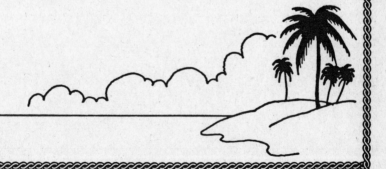

As we continue our pinpointing of the particular foods that merit honorable mention for keeping Hawaiians and other Polynesians at the peak of good health, we discover foods with special advantages.

In this chapter, we present foods that are:

EASILY DIGESTED

VALUED BABY FOOD

NON-ALLERGENIC

HIGH IN NUTRITION

LONGEVITY RELATED

RICH IN TRACE MINERALS

SOURCE OF CALCIUM

DIGESTIVE AID

HEALTHFUL GELATIN

AID TO NORMAL ELIMINATION

HIGH IN PROTEIN

BEAUTY DRINK

NON-FAT PROTEIN

BODY BUILDING

NERVE TONIC

HEALTHFUL THROUGH FERMENTATION

PROTEIN BOOSTER

RICH IN ENZYMES

ALKALINE IN REACTION

LOW-CALORIE

SLIMMING

HOME GROWABLE

ORGANIC

SOURCE OF VITAMIN A

NATURAL PRESERVATIVE

ENERGY RESTORING

ANTACID

The eating habits of modern day Hawaiians and other Polynesians contribute to their longevity now. Some of these are based on island traditions. Others are newly acquired, through their introduction by the arrival of peoples from Pacific rim countries, but are nonetheless important as health factors.

The introduction of new foods by people from other countries is an ongoing process all over the world. When electricity arrived in Bali recently, vendors of cold soft drinks appeared overnight. Pizza, an old favorite in Italy, is a relatively new food in the United States. Japan is currently undergoing a shift from rice to pizza, French bread and hamburger buns.

The trend is so rapid in Japan that the consumption of traditional rice has dropped 30 percent in the last 15 years. In order to get rid of the surplus, the Japanese government is pushing new products like rice coffee made from parched rice, rice juice which is said to have a flavor similar to pineapple, and even rice wine. Bakers who have switched to Western flour for their bread are being compelled to mix in a percentage of rice flour.

So, as we survey eating habits in Hawai'i and the South Pacific today, going beyond the fruits and nuts reviewed in the last chapter, we begin to see the effects of many cultures. However, we are going to begin with a food that is typically Hawaiian and Polynesian.

THE HAWAIIAN AND POLYNESIAN "STAFF OF LIFE"

Taro is one of the oldest known vegetables. In Egyptian history, *taro* was mentioned as early as 23 B.C., although under a different name. According to ancient records, it was taken to Italy. *Taro* was later found in Sri Lanka (formerly Ceylon), Malay and India. When the first Europeans arrived in Japan and in New Zealand, they found *taro* already under cultivation.

Taro is not native to Hawai'i. The Polynesian voyagers carried it aboard their double-hull sailing canoes. They knew that, cooked and crushed, with no water added, it could be wrapped in *ti* leaves and kept for several months.

Historians estimate that *taro* was brought to Hawai'i around 450 A.D. In the early days, some varieties of *taro* were used strictly as offerings to the Hawaiian gods. Others were only allowed for the *ali'i*, or chiefs. But that still left enough *taro* to make it the mainstay of the Hawaiian diet.

Early Hawaiians are said to have eaten from 10 to 15 pounds of this staple a day. It is credited for providing them with their sturdy bone structure and beautiful teeth.

When the *taro* root is pounded and water is added, the resulting "pudding" is called *poi*. The thickness is measured by the ease with which it can be eaten with the fingers. Some people like two-finger *poi*, some like three-finger *poi*.

Mainlanders can now buy *poi* in jars and in powdered form. In the old days the plant had many medicinal uses which are not available to mainlanders because they involved the whole *taro* plant. The cut leaf was rubbed onto insect bites to take away the sting. The juice of the stalk, blended with sugar or coconut milk, was drunk to reduce fever. The cut root was used as a styptic to halt bleeding.

Taro leaves and *poi* are served at every *lu'au* in Hawai'i, and in every restaurant that serves Hawaiian food. Both are available in supermarkets on the main islands of the Hawaiian chain. Most of it is grown in the island of Kaua'i, but there are *taro* patches on every island, even the bustling island of O'ahu.

EASILY DIGESTED; VALUED BABY FOOD. Because of its small starch grains, *poi* is easily digested. It is, therefore, an excellent food for people with certain health problems involving the digestion, such as ulcers. It is an excellent baby food for this reason, and you will find it in jars in the baby food section of your grocery store or supermarket.

NON-ALLERGENIC. Doctors see in *poi* a food that is practically non-allergenic. Dr. Albert H. Rowe, a noted allergy specialist, is quoted as saying, "The most commonly eaten grains produce most allergies. In America, wheat is the chief offender. In Japan, it is rice." A noted allergy specialist in Hawai'i, Dr. L. Q. Pang, has stated, *"Poi* is one of the foods we usually recommend to patients with food allergies. Through our experience, if a patient has proved allergic to certain grains, chances are they can eat *poi* with no adverse reaction."

HIGH IN NUTRITION. Nutritionally speaking, *poi* has less calories than its equivalent in rice or potatoes. It is lower in protein than either but far exceeds both in iron, calcium and the vitamin B-complex ingredients, thiamine and riboflavin.

The taste of *poi* is controversial. Visitors to Hawai'i liken it to wallpaper paste, but that is because their eyes tell them ahead of time that it looks like, and therefore should taste like, chocolate mousse.

It doesn't. It doesn't even come close. But many who develop a taste for *poi* make it a life-long habit, and live a longer life for it.

For kids, add freeze-dried *poi* to milk with a dash of vanilla. As a frozen delight, combine *poi,* sugar and milk in a heavy consistency. Place in an ice tray, insert toothpicks and freeze.

If you have difficulty locating ready-to-eat *poi* in jars, the dehydrated *poi* in jars, or the freeze-dried "instant" *poi* in envelopes, write to this company for information: *Poi* Co., Ltd., 1603 Republican St., Honolulu, Hawaii 96819.

The leaves of the *taro* plant, properly washed and soaked, are like a delectable spinach. But you will have to come to the islands to enjoy them.

LONGEVITY RELATED. Seiyo H. is 83 years old. He loves nature. He works as a farmer all day long in the same fields where he labored as a young man. He works just as vigorously as when he was young, too. Can you see Seiyo with his straw hat and boots, surrounded by the fluted Koʻolau mountains in Oʻahu, embellished with waterfalls? Can you tell what crop he is harvesting? Seiyo is a *taro* farmer. His *taro* is grown in running water, somewhat like rice. He is still able to harvest ten bags of the *taro* corm a week, pulling up the plant, chopping off the tops and replanting the tops to keep the field in production.

Although Seiyo works hard at 83, *taro* has furnished him with an income to raise his family and it has obviously kept him in the best of health.

VALUABLE VEGETABLES FROM THE SEA

Before the advent of health food stores, people all over the world, even in remote inland areas, considered the ocean as a prime source of nutritional food.

According to Oriental tradition, the sea is the starting point for man's biological evolution. The Chinese characters for the word "sea" are a combination of "water" and "mother." Both the Chinese and the Japanese have a great respect for sea-grasses and plants, a respect shared by the Polynesians with whom they came to live.

Several kinds of seaweed, more properly called sea-vegetables, are in everyday use in Hawaiʻi. Some are still known by their Hawaiian names; others, because they are common in Japan, are known by Japanese names.

The umbrella term for seaweed in Hawaiian is *limu*. Each kind of *limu* was given its own name, usually referring to its flower-like appearance *(lehua)* or its location *(lipe'epe'e,* meaning hidden).

Common Japanese varieties are *hiziki, nori* and *kanten,* the last type being commonly known in the West as *agar agar.* Other Western terms for these same vegetables of the sea are kelp and dulse.

RICH IN TRACE MINERALS. Seaweed is one of the best known sources of the trace minerals potassium and magnesium and is a good source of iodine. The vitamin C content is equivalent to that of many fruits and vegetables. Other vitamins in abundant supply in seaweeds are A, B_1, B_2, B_{12}, thiamine, niacin and D.

SOURCE OF CALCIUM. Seaweeds are also rich in calcium, and *hiziki,* a stringy black sea grass that grows on submerged rocky ledges, has 14 times as much calcium as milk—14 milligrams per gram, compared to milk's 1 milligram per gram. Calcium is essential for teeth and bones, as well as for the nervous system.

DIGESTIVE AID. Like other sources of vitality, seaweeds contain the marginal question mark that defies chemical analysis. For instance, they are known to develop healthy intestinal flora which aid in digestion, similar to the way that clabbered milk, such as acidophilus, implants strains of bacteria that help digestion.

Why is it that foods that are good for us lack taste appeal? *Poi* and seaweed are in the same ballpark. And it is quite a different ballpark from the one where ice cream and candy are found (although seaweed has been used as a filler for ice cream for decades).

Actually, our tastes have been subverted. Sugar has been the subverting agent. Sweetness has clouded all the subtle tastes of nature to which we were once privy. You will find no sweet desserts in Hawaiian, Japanese or Chinese restaurants or homes. If you enjoy Hawaiian *haupia,* made from coconut and arrowroot, rest assured that there is little, if any, sugar. If you enjoy Japanese *yokan,* made from red beans and *kanten (agar agar),* again there is little sweetening. If you enjoy Chinese almond jelly, it is made from powdered almonds and *kanten* and little, if any, sweetening.

Western tastes are perverted tastes, with sugar acting as the great hypnotizer of the taste buds: "Use me to make all things taste good." If the taste is not sweet, the taste is not good.

We can de-hypnotize and recondition our taste buds to detect the subtle delicacy of natural foods. We can develop a taste for seaweed.

The best way to start is to add seaweed to different recipes. It goes well with land vegetables. It makes a tangy complement to salads and stews. See Chapter 11 for recipe ideas.

HOW TO OBTAIN SEAWEED WITHOUT GETTING YOUR FEET WET

A familiar sight a generation ago was a small group of Hawaiian women dressed in *mu'umu'us* and straw hats, cleaning *limu* along a beach.

You can still see a lone figure on a beach in Hawai'i, knee deep in the ocean, gathering *limu.* He or she will probably clean it, take it home and cook it for dinner with fish and *poi,* thus perpetuating the staple meal of old Hawai'i.

It is still as valid a meal today as it was then, nutritionally speaking, containing all the necessary protein, carbohydrates, fats, minerals and vitamins for healthful nutrition.

But it is now a lot easier to obtain seaweed.

Kanten, commonly called *agar agar* in the West, is actually a gelatin made from varieties of seaweed. It is available in Oriental food markets and health food stores.

One of the principle seaweeds in *kanten* is *tengusa,* which means "grass from heaven" in Japanese. Its botanical name is *gelidium.* A short sea grass with a slender beard-like stem and leaves, it grows several feet deep along most of the coastline of Japan. It grows to maturity in nine months, budding in the fall and being harvested in the summer.

Let's look in on its processing. This is done in remote mountain areas where the temperatures are cold enough as required for the final stages. After being soaked to take away salt and sand, the seaweed is simmered in a large iron kettle overnight. It begins to melt and the water in the kettle becomes thick and soapy.

In the morning it is strained and poured into shallow rectangular wooden boxes lined in long rows. Within an hour it hardens into a heavy gelatin. It is then cut into bars or strips and spread out on bamboo mats exposed to air and sun. Some mountain valleys in Nagano and Gifu, Japan become white as if blanketed with snow, so covered are they with the drying *kanten*.

While drying and airing in this way, the *kanten* turns from slightly pink to colorless and translucent and it loses all the odor brought with it from the sea. At night the *kanten* freezes and moisture comes out of suspension in the gelatin, forming an icy glace on the surface. In the morning, this melts and runs off into the field. This process keeps purifying and condensing the *kanten*. Finally, only a flaky, brittle celluloid-like product remains.

HEALTHFUL GELATIN. We recommend the *kanten* made this way naturally (as by Muso Co., Ltd.), rather than that made with chemical softening agents and bleaches. It has no odor and is a healthful all-purpose gelatin.

AID TO NORMAL ELIMINATION. One health advantage of *kanten* you may notice is that it relaxes the intestines, promoting normal elimination.

Hiziki is perhaps the best known sea vegetable. It grows on Japan's southern Pacific coast. It is found closer to the water surface and is thus easily gathered. Harvested in the spring, its tough texture necessitates cooking overnight before being dried in the sun, the only processing needed. When you cook *hiziki*, it becomes tender and chewy like pasta.

If you cannot find *hiziki* in your local health food store or the Oriental department of your supermarket, you can obtain it by mail from Erewhon Natural Food, 342 Newbury St., Boston, Massachusetts 02115.

HIGH IN PROTEIN. They are also a supplier of *nori*, which has a protein content that surpasses the water and fat reduced protein content of beef, beating it 35 percent to 25 percent, surpassing even the remarkable soybean, which has 34 percent protein.

The fact that we have highlighted the Japanese varieties takes no credit away from other seaweeds. The Japanese varieties are one of the health secrets of the Hawaiians and other Polynesians.

Kelp and dulse are just as valuable as sources of fiber, iodine and micronutrients of the sea. Their fine processing into fine powder and flakes may detract somewhat from the vitamin content, but the greatest value of seaweeds is in their mineral content and that is only minimally affected.

One large Canadian supplier offers kelp flakes, kelp granules and kelp powder. Dulse is offered in flakes and powder. Atlantic Mariculture Limited is located in Dartmouth, Nova Scotia, Canada B2W 344.

THE BEAN THAT DOES A STEAK'S JOB

Meat prices are going up. Not enough cattle are coming to the market to fill the increasing demand for beef. Overpopulation and over-grazed grasslands may eventually make beef a rare food like caviar.

Beef is produced in Hawai'i. Ranching is a major industry on the Big Island. However, beef is not a Hawaiian and Polynesian health secret. About the only advantage there is to eating Hawaiian beef over mainland beef is that there is less likelihood that artificial means are being used to fatten the herds.

If beef should disappear altogether, local people might miss the beef stew and the hamburgers but they would not suffer from protein deficiency.

The reason is the soybean. The soybean is indeed one of Hawai'i's health secrets.

You do not often see the soybean served as such (as baked beans), but it is usually converted into *shoyu*, *tofu* and *miso*.

In the summer of 1978, 70 people met in Ann Arbor, Michigan, to establish the Soycrafters Association of North America (SANA). The non-profit organization will facilitate communications between the over 100 firms producing soy products such as *shoyu* sauce, *tofu*, *miso* and soy milk. *Tofu* shops and soy dairies are now established in over 30 states. To find the one closest to you, write SANA, Box 76, Bodega, California 94922.

As we begin to describe these soy products to you, starting with *tofu*, you may wish to make your own. Making *tofu* is easier than baking bread. A *tofu* kit, complete with a 16-page booklet of instructions and recipes, a mahogany setting box, pressing sack, cheesecloth and enough natural *Nigari* solidifier for ten batches of *tofu* can also be obtained from Bodega, California. Write to The Learning Tree, Box 76.

Perhaps the first American to learn the secret of the soybean was Paul C. Bragg, whom we have already mentioned. When he was an associate editor of Bernarr Macfadden's famous *Physical Culture Maga-*

zine in the 1920's, it was decided that it would be valuable to research the touted energy, vitality and health of the Manchurian people. It was an arduous journey in those days, but well worth the discovery Bragg made: soy milk.

BEAUTY DRINK. Bragg found the beautiful Manchurian women drinking soy milk and eating the solids from the soy milk. Manchurian men maintained their virility and working productivity into what we call old age, by eating these products of soy milk.

Bragg saw the Manchurians make soy milk by grinding soybeans that had been soaked in water for 24 hours and then straining it through cheesecloth. The rough part was fed to the animals. The liquid soy milk was then cooked with gypsum (calcium sulfate) to precipitate the solids. These solids that dropped to the bottoms of the containers were pressed, and the resulting product was bean curd. It is called *dom foo yuen* in Chinese, *tofu* in Japanese.

The soybeans themselves seem to ask that some processing be done. They cannot be eaten raw, as they contain a digestive inhibitor which blocks the working of the enzyme trypsin. Soaked and then cooked, they are edible and nutritious.

NON-FAT PROTEIN. Most protein sources contain animal fat. Beef, veal, lamb, pork, game, poultry and dairy products carry a price tag on their protein in the form of artery-clogging cholesterol. Fish and seafood are good sources of protein and they cost less. Soybeans are even better, with no animal fat price to pay.

Mainland use of soybeans is similar to that of other dried beans. Housewives buy the boxes of dried soybeans just as they do lentils or other dried beans. They soak them in much the same way (although the water needs to be changed twice with soy), and then they bake them, perhaps in a casserole with tomato sauce.

This is fine, but it is limiting in two ways. First, it limits the many tastes of soy. Second, it limits its scope for providing nutrition.

Soybean crop production in the United States went from less than 2,000,000 acres in 1924 to 56,000,000 acres in 1973, exceeding even wheat and corn with its nine-billion-dollar value. Are American housewives making casseroles or chilis with that many cans and boxes of soybeans? Are 500,000,000 pounds of soybeans being poured from nonappetizing cans or soaked overnight each year in the United States, when the taste of this sloppy orange stuff is definitely on the minus side of the scale?

The answer is no. The beans are being pressed for their oil and the rest is being fed to animals.

But now a secret of the Orient, known for decades in Hawai'i, is being murmured across the land: *tofu*.

There are reports that sales of *tofu* are doubling in the United States every six months and that the volume is now approaching 100,000 pounds a day.

Tofu is a soybean curd sold in white blocks. It can be mashed and added to tuna dishes, chopped fine and added to omelets, sliced and fried for serving with meat and vegetables.

BODY BUILDING. However you eat it, you gain in protein and calcium, two essential building blocks of the body. Soy protein is complete protein with all eight of the essential amino acids. In fact, it has been called one of the most nourishing body building foods in the world. It is thus an excellent food for children.

NERVE TONIC. Tofu also has a high lecithin content, and is therefore helpful for mental fatigue and as a nerve tonic. Since lecithin also helps the body rid itself of excess cholesterol, this soybean product not only supplies no cholesterol but can actually lower cholesterol levels.

Tofu is an easy way to enjoy soybeans, a not too enjoyable food. *Tofu* is tasty, adaptable for a variety of uses, and good for you.

A HIGH PROTEIN SEASONING

HEALTHFUL THROUGH FERMENTATION. Another derivative of the soybean is *miso*. It is a fermented product of the soybean with all of its high protein, high calcium and high nutritive values, plus one more: *lactobacillus*.

Throughout recorded history, peoples with records of good health and longevity have always had fermented products in their diets, such as yogurt or apple cider vinegar. There appear to be beneficial bacteria that help us to digest and assimilate the nutrients in food. The *lactobacillus* is one.

It would be hard for most Japanese to live without *miso*. Its subtle aromatic flavor is so basic to the Japanese diet that it has become for them synonymous with mother and home. The Japanese mother uses *miso* in soups, vegetables, sauces, dressings and spreads.

Paste-like in appearance and texture, *miso* is prepared by mixing soybeans with salt and usually another cereal grain. After cooking, a mold called *koji* is added and the mixture is placed in cedar kegs under the weight of heavy stones. There it is allowed to ferment for at least one year.

PROTEIN BOOSTER. This fermenting process breaks down the soybeans and grains so that their nutrients are quickly and easily digestible. The protein structure is disassembled into 18 different amino acids so that even other foods consumed at the same meal, which are missing some essential amino acids, will become complete proteins thanks to the *miso*.

RICH IN ENZYMES. Fermentation also produces a wealth of enzymes that help with the digestive process for all the rest of your meal.

ALKALINE IN REACTION. Miso is quite alkaline in its reaction, thus assisting digestion in still another way.

LOW-CALORIE. The favorite Japanese use of *miso* is to make *miso* soup. Even in Hawai'i, many families of Japanese descent still awaken to the smell of *miso* soup which, with rice, is considered a meal in itself— even for breakfast. An 8-ounce bowl of nourishing *miso* soup contains only 36 calories.

However, for Western tastes, *miso* can be used in any soup as you would use a rich meat stock, and similarly in stews. Use *miso* as you would use ketchup or Worcestershire in sauces and dressings, cheese in casseroles and spreads, and chutney or relish for a condiment.

In short, it is an all-purpose seasoning, thickener and condiment that, unlike most seasonings, thickeners and condiments, actually goes to work to build your body for a longer, healthier life.

If you cannot find *miso* in your supermarket or health food store, look in your telephone book's yellow pages under Chinese or Japanese food products.

A HIGH PROTEIN SAUCE

On every table in every Chinese restaurant in the mainland United States is a small vial or bottle of soy sauce.

In Hawai'i, this is found in practically every household.

Shoyu, tamari or soy sauce is another fermented product of the soybean. It contains most of the basic health advantages just described. It is a fast-spreading health secret of Hawai'i and the Orient.

Japanese *shoyu* is said to have graced the table of Louis XIV. The naming of the bean *"soya"* was said to have been done by an 18th century Swedish botanist trying to pronounce *shoyu,* the product made from it.

The term *tamari* is used interchangeably with *shoyu*, but *tamari* is actually a different soy product. If you buy *tamari* in the United States stores, it is *shoyu*. But when Japanese sources begin exporting the real *tamari*, some confusion is expected to take place.

Meanwhile, *tamari, shoyu* or soy sauce is made from soybeans, wheat, salt and water. First the soybeans are steamed until they are soft enough to be easily crushed with the fingers but still firm enough to retain their shape. Simultaneously, the wheat is roasted in hot sand until it turns brown in color and has a fragrant aroma. To the soybeans and wheat is then added the fermenting agent *koji*.

What follows is a complicated process of storage, removal of molds and further storage and processing. After it is fully aged, the solids are drained off and the liquid is heated at 176 degrees Fahrenheit for one hour, long enough to terminate the bacterial action without harming the valuable enzymes in the *shoyu*. It is then bottled for your table.

A dash of *shoyu* in vegetables, soups or stews is a dash of taste and a dash of nutrition. It can be used in basting, broiling, baking, boiling and sauteeing.

Shoyu is affected adversely by sunlight and heat, so it is sold in a dark glass bottle but should still be kept in a shaded place, well away from the range heating units.

HIGH IN PROTEIN; SOURCE OF CALCIUM. Think of *shoyu* as the soybean itself—a storehouse of protein, calcium and other nutrients. Keep it in your kitchen, convenient to both the range and the dining table.

Begin to use *shoyu*. Experiment on different dishes. It not only adds taste, but draws out the distinctive taste of what you are cooking. It is a healthful sauce ingredient. It is a healthful spice—the spice of life.

Another good source for sea vegetable and soybean products, if you cannot find them at your local Oriental grocery or health food store, is Westbrae Natural Foods, 4240 Hollis St., Emeryville, California 94608.

THE MEANING OF GREEN TO HAWAIIAN AND POLYNESIAN PEOPLES

SLIMMING. Two scientists at the University of Illinois recently made some interesting computations. They figured that if the 100,000,000 adult Americans who are overweight would cut down on their caloric intake, slim down and stay slim, enough energy would be saved in planting, cultivating, harvesting, processing, storing, transporting and selling the food that keeps them plump to supply the electrical requirements of Boston, Chicago, Washington and San Francisco.

But, as we see it, if they learned about a certain Hawaiian and Polynesian health secret, they would not cut down on intake, but merely switch, and so no energy would be saved while they slimmed down.

It takes just as much energy to grow, harvest and transport slenderizing green vegetables as it does sugar, flour, potatoes and other fattening foods.

There is hardly a diet that does not permit eating all the salad and leafy vegetables you want. Nutritionists know that salad materials and leafy vegetables are high in nutrition and low in calories.

But the people of the Pacific islands know something else—the greener, the better.

It is not necessarily chlorophyll, the chief factor that makes a plant green, that explains why a dark green leafy vegetable is better than a whitish green one. But the presence of chlorophyll signals the presence of other nutrients.

Many ancient people believed in the nascent life force of spring. As the hibernating earth warms, green returns in the willow, grass and shrub buds. They saw green as the healing color. And they saw greens as the "healthier food."

HIGH NUTRITION. Compare the color of the local brands of lettuce the next time you are in Hawai'i with the mainland brands. Here the best seller is green *Manoa*; the loser is white iceberg lettuce.

Compare the colors of the different varieties of lettuce in your local supermarket. Switch to the greener types for your money's worth in nutrition.

Compare the color of your leafy vegetables, using green as a gauge.

Switch to beet tops, spinach, dandelion greens and other deep green varieties.

The Chinese have always been especially appreciative of greens. Chinese cabbage in Hawai'i seems greener than the Chinese cabbage we have seen with increasing frequency in mainland supermarkets. Still, we would recommend that you investigate Chinese vegetables like *won bok* (cabbage) and snow peas. The latter are available frozen everywhere, but inquire at your local Chinese restaurant to see if there is a local supplier of the fresh produce.

Keep your antenna up for edible green leaves. To list the minerals and vitamins in these vegetables would be like throwing the whole book at you. Hawaiians and other Polynesians have been loving greens forever. But they are different greens. One example, *taro* leaves, as we said before, is just not available on the U. S. mainland. Neither are other local favorites.

But you have your own storehouse of greens, thanks to nature's beneficence. You have watercress and parsley. You have brussels sprouts and kale.

Those of you who live in rural areas have the advantage of wild greens, free for the picking. Dandelion greens, lambs quarters and wild onions are examples.

City folk can grow watercress, mint and onion grass in their kitchens and window boxes.

HOME GROWABLE. Here is one Hawaiian leafy green you can also grow: sweet potato leaves. Yes, sweet potato leaves are not only edible, but they are delicious and nutritious. Here's how to grow them: Cut off the top section of the tuber and place it in a jar, with water, in a dark place until sprouts begin to form. Then place it in the light. After several days put it into sunlight. When enough leaves have formed, you can harvest them. Steam them for a tasty healthful vegetable, or pick the tips for your salads.

SPROUTING BETTER HEALTH

You can also grow your own sprouts.

Stuart W. visited Hawai'i a number of times and was impressed by the variety of sprouts that were always available in the markets—soybean sprouts, alfalfa sprouts, mung bean sprouts, and so on.

One day, financial disaster threatened him and his family of seven.

For six months their food bill totaled $52.50. At today's prices that would probably be equivalent to $100.00. But that is still incredible for 180 days of three meals a day for seven people.

Stuart's solution was sprouts. Sprouts played a large role in their diet. "No sickness, no colds, no flu or other problems affected any of us," he reports.

ORGANIC. Anyone can grow sprouts. It is foolproof. No worry about soil conditions or spraying against pests. Cheap, organic, vital, fresh vegetables are yours for the asking.

The procedure is to soak your seeds or dried beans overnight in just enough water to cover them. A mason jar or wide-mouthed bottle is best. In the morning, drain, rinse and place the jar in a tilt with a porous covering like a paper towel, cheesecloth or a piece of sheer nylon. Several times during the day, pour water into the jar, shake gently and pour off, again laying the jar at an angle. Keep the jar away from direct sunlight.

SOURCE OF VITAMIN A. Sprouts usually double in nutrition on the second day and are ready to eat soon after. But their bulk and nutrition keep increasing. After four or five days, you can put the sprouts in bright sunlight for an hour or two to develop that bright green color indicative of vitamin A and chlorophyll—and they're ready for your evening meal.

AN ANTACID FROM JAPAN

One of the Hawaiian and Polynesian health secrets is still a secret even in Hawai'i. We would like to share this secret of secrets before we close this chapter on those foods that contribute to youthfulness and vibrant health on these islands.

As we write, there is in our refrigerator a small plastic container of something that looks like an undergrown apricot. Actually, it is a dried plum called *umeboshi*.

The *ume*, or Japanese plum, is used as both a medicine and a food. It is usually picked in June before it is fully ripe, and then packed in vats with crude salt. Next, *shiso* leaves are placed over the plums in the vat. Known in America as "beef steak plant," *shiso* supplies the reddish color of *umeboshi*.

NATURAL PRESERVATIVE. Shiso also contains a natural preservative called perilla-aldehyde that is said to have a thousand times the strength of synthetic preservatives without their risks and contra-indications.

By mid-July, the plums are ready for the drying process out in the hot sun. But first they are returned overnight to the vats to absorb more of their own vinegar. It is this liquid plum vinegar that is the source of the medicinal properties. At first it has a sharp acidity; then it turns sour.

Modern methods are being developed to hasten the production of *umeboshi,* but suppliers like Muso, mentioned earlier in this chapter, stick to the organic, traditional ways.

ENERGY RESTORING. The citric acid in *umeboshi* is said to help with the elimination of lactic acid from the body. Lactic acid is a cause of fatigue.

ANTACID. Umeboshi causes an alkaline reaction when digested and is thus a popular antacid. Eating just one or two of the sour plums can help with digestion. Pregnant women who have a desire for foods with a sour flavor enjoy *umeboshi.*

The nutritious plum sits unobtrusively on the Japanese foodstuff shelves in Hawai'i. We doubt that even your health food store carries them. But you can find the closest source by writing to Erewhon in Boston, at the address supplied earlier in this chapter.

Now for some of the more "open" health secrets of Hawaiians and Polynesians.

7

*Polynesian
Health Practices
That Work Anywhere*

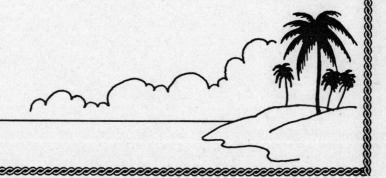

In this chapter we examine the basic elements of healthful living: fresh air, fresh water and sleep.

Although Hawai'i and Polynesia are environmentally endowed with many blessings not available to mainlanders, there are ways to improve present conditions where you live.

In the process of comparing this Pacific area and your home environment, some positive steps that you can take become apparent. These involve, among others, the following:

PURIFYING BREATH TECHNIQUE

POSITIVE THOUGHTS

A BETTER PARK

REDUCING EXPOSURE TO SMOKERS

BARRING FUMES

IONIZING YOUR AIR

SPECIAL BENEFITS OF A SHOWER

IMPROVED OXYGEN DELIVERY

PURER WATER

SPRING WATER

DISTILLED WATER

NEUTRAL SOFT DRINKS

A BETTER BEER

ALCOHOLIC PROTEIN

LOW-CALORIE THIRST QUENCHER

FRESH AIR HOLIDAYS

AIR PURIFYING PLANTS

TOXIN PREVENTIVE DETOURS

SOFTENED WATER

WASHED FOOD

THE BEST SLEEP

NATURAL "SLEEPING PILL"

NIGHT AIR

- Breathe fresh air.
- Drink fresh water.
- Get plenty of sleep.

These are health axioms, not health secrets.

Still, Hawaiians and other Polynesian people have adopted ways to apply these basic principles because they contribute to an excellent track record in healthful living.

As we leave off on our discussion of foods and get into activities, we recognize that there is a tendency on the part of most people to make short shrift of this aspect of physical health.

"Did you say sprouts? Fantastic! How do I make them?"

"Did you say deep breaths? Ridiculous! I'll breathe the way I always breathe."

Some people feel this way even about foods. They are so stuck in their ways that a health secret from the moon would not move them.

Paul V., who sends about 60 workers in small boats into the waters off Plymouth, Massachusetts to harvest a half ton of seaweed a day, was in his truck filled with seaweed when a woman asked him if he was cleaning the beach. When Paul explained how seaweed is used in ice cream and chocolate milk as well as being a food itself, she replied, "Who do you think you are, trying to make a fool out of me?"

Some of the subtle changes in the way you live, which we will be describing as Polynesian health secrets in this chapter, may appear so childish to you that you, too, may be tempted to say, "Are you trying to make a fool out of me?"

No, we are not. We are sharing valid health practices, as childish as they may sound. Polynesians, no matter what their ages, are like children. And have you ever seen an old or senile child?

VITAL ENERGY AND ITS CONTROL BY BREATH

Science is just beginning to experiment with life energy. It has only recently been recognized in the scientific world as a real energy, despite its acknowledgment in just about every culture.

Whether we are talking about *orenda* with an American Indian, *mana* with a Hawaiian, or *prana* with a guru from India, we are talking about a very real universal life force that we could all use more of.

Each culture has its own way of increasing the flow of this vital energy. Max Freedom Long, in *Secret Science Behind Miracles*, a book devoted to the work of the *kahunas* of Hawai'i, described how the laying on of hands to heal another on many occasions brought a return flow of negative energy such as that derived from nicotine or alcohol. When an intoxicated man was touched, the healer became intoxicated and the drunk man sobered up.

This same effect has been seen "on camera" through Kirlian photography. Dr. Milton Trager of Honolulu, founder of a mind-body therapy called Tragering, had Dr. Thelma Moss of California take Kirlian photographs of his and his patient's hands before and after administering the therapy. It distinctly showed a reduced vital energy in his hands, and an increased vital energy in the hands of the recipient.

Hawaiians use the hands in the transfer of vital energy and we will go into this later. But they also have a solo procedure to increase their vital energy. It is done through the breath.

Perhaps you will understand the vital importance of this energy and the scientific miracles it can accomplish if you play a simple parlor game that has been around for decades.

A person sits in a chair. Four other people attempt to lift the chair with him or her in it. If it can be done easily, then the number of fingers that may be used are reduced so that it becomes impossible. If a light person is in the chair, maybe only two fingers of each hand may be used. Once it is determined that the four people cannot lift the chair with that amount of fingers, you are ready to demonstrate the effect of breath. All five inhale deeply together several times, then hold their breath and lift. The seated person will be lifted.

Long tells of experiments by Dr. Hereward Carrington, one-time dean of psychical researchers, who played this game using platform scales and recorded a drop in total weight at the moment of lifting from 700 down to 650 total pounds.

The ancient Hawaiians who ran long distances carrying messages for the high chiefs used a breathing discipline that gave them superior speed and endurance.

PURIFYING BREATH TECHNIQUE. Kahunas used breath-holding techniques to help their patients recover from illness. One such technique is known as the "HA" breath. It is done by inhaling slowly to the count of three, holding to the count of six, and then expelling the air forcefully. Some people loudly exclaim, "HA!" as they expel the air. It is believed by some that the name HA-wai'i is derived from this breath that manipulates vital energy.

Hannah Veary, a respected teacher of ancient healing arts in Hawai'i, reported seeing broken ends of bone move into place as the HA breath was breathed into a cupped hand which was passed over the damaged area.

Do not repeat these breaths more than a total of three times. Be sure the air is fresh where you are, and avoid doing it in places such as on a sidewalk where heavy traffic is passing.

As you exhale with a loud "HA," feel that you are expelling all poisons and foreign matter from your body. As you inhale, feel that you are taking in vital energy that is being distributed to all cells of your body.

Donald L. got the "Polynesian paralysis" shortly after moving his family from Knoxville, Tennessee, to Honolulu. This is the term given to a lethargy that comes over just about everybody who visits Hawai'i. You just don't feel like doing anything but lying under a palm tree and taking in the beauty. It usually passes in a few days, but in Donald's case, it lasted for weeks until we told him about the HA breath. He did it three times on awakening and on the second day he was so full of energy to do all the things that needed doing, he became a beehive of activity and the doldrums were forgotten—permanently.

THE REAL MEANING BEHIND FIJIAN FIRE WALKING

The scene is the Andrews Amphitheater at the University of Hawaii. A fire pit that was started hours ago is approached by two physicists. They read a special thermometer and announce that the temperature is 1200 degrees Fahrenheit and the stones are red hot. The audience waits expectantly.

Then there is chanting. A long file of Fijians approach, dressed in traditional costume. They circle the fire pit. Then they step onto the stones and continue their slow walk in the pit. Some pick up the red hot stones and fling them aside defiantly. In about five minutes the Fijian fire walk has ended and there is not a burn to be found among the group, not even a blister.

We do not mean to oversimplify the explanation of how this is done, for this ritual has a long history of development. A few of our friends have been indoctrinated into the method, whereby they are confident in the knowledge that they can walk on hot stones, and they were able to do it, too. In one case, a man wondered momentarily why he was not feeling the heat. Instantly, he felt it, and had to hop off to the side and out of the pit. His feet were seriously blistered.

This is psychosomatic illness in reverse. Doctors now know that attitudes and emotions cause most illnesses. We are beginning to find out that attitudes and emotions can be used to prevent illness and injury as well.

Few of us have the mental discipline of the Fijian firewalkers, so do not expect that you could walk on hot coals and not be burned. But all of us have the ability to think negatively and invite problems, or to think positively and invite solutions.

The *kahunas* almost always accompanied their herbal and other cures with the admonition, "Never again think of your ailment."

This is the real meaning behind the fire walking.

POSITIVE THOUGHTS. No matter what your physical problem or disease, never accept it as a part of you. When it has been relieved, never think about it again.

Consider yourself to be perfectly healthy, despite any detours. Consider all imperfections as temporary and not really belonging to you.

This may seem to be a childlike philosophy, but it works. Your mind has an important role to play in running your body.

HOW TO FRESHEN THE AIR YOU BREATHE

The sky in Hawai'i is not gray. It is blue—deep blue. To the people of some United States cities, a blue sky is about as frequent as a blue moon. The reason why the Hawaiian sky is so blue is that the air is clean and fresh. The reason why the air is clean and fresh is that trade winds blow the exhaust fumes from cars, trucks, buses and planes out to sea.

According to a recent check by the Environmental Protection

Agency, Honolulu has the cleanest air of all urban areas with a population over 200,000. In fact, it was the only city in that bracket that stayed within acceptable levels for *all* pollutants, including vehicle exhausts.

It is no secret that fresh Hawaiian air contributes to the longevity of the people who live in Hawai'i. But there are ways in which the people here protect the air they breathe. Some of these methods are not available to you, like being outdoors a lot and keeping windows wide open most of the time. But you can still move a little further in that direction.

A BETTER PARK. Most parks in Hawai'i are by the sea. But there are some inland that are away from heavily trafficked roads. You may want to change the parks you are frequenting, sacrificing proximity for air purity.

It is estimated that, every day of your life, you take about 2000 gallons of air into your lungs. From that air, your body extracts oxygen. But whatever else is in the air can also wind up in your body.

REDUCING EXPOSURE TO SMOKERS. Smoke from tobacco, gas and chemical pollutants is taking its toll on American health. Strict laws have been passed in Hawai'i governing smoking in public places.

BARRING FUMES. No matter how hot the day, motorists in Hawai'i will close their windows in heavy traffic, especially if there is a fume-spewing bus alongside them.

According to the Ion Foundation, manufacturers of "Energaire," an interesting experiment was performed having to do with ionized air. Laboratory animals were placed in a chamber. The air was ionized. Even though all of the oxygen was used up, the animals remained energetic and alert. When the reverse situation was created—no ions but plenty of oxygen—the animals became drowsy, irritable and sluggish.

Ions are small, electrically charged particles in the air. They are constantly being formed in three basic ways:

1. The sun generates trillions of them every day, renewing the protective ozone layer and the ionosphere that envelop our atmosphere.
2. Oceans, forests and waterfalls are constantly revitalizing the air with these ions.
3. Lightning creates ions.

All three of these ion-generating factors are taking place in Hawai'i, but one of them is probably happening more frequently in your part of the country, at least during certain months of the year. That's number 3—lightning. The scarcity of ions created by electrical storms in Hawai'i, however, is more than made up for by the sun and the plant life.

IONIZING YOUR AIR. De-ionized air is dead air. Most air conditioning systems remove ions from the air. But there is a way to add ions to your air.

Air ionizers are now available. If you are feeling tired and worn out, you might try adding an electrical charge to your environment. Test yourself before and after a storm. If you feel uncomfortable and irritable before a storm and then feel relieved, even exhilarated after a storm, you may need an air ionizer, at home, at work or both.

Before a storm, there is a build-up of positively charged air ions. These are not what the body seeks. After a storm, there is a preponderance of negatively charged ions, usually oxygen atoms. These help our bodies to utilize oxygen and, by so doing, they lift up our energy and our spirits.

Negative ions have the added advantage of helping to precipitate dust, pollen, smoke and germs out of the air, leaving the air in a living room or office cleaner and fresher—closer to island air.

Desert winds create a positive ion count which makes people feel uncomfortable and drained of energy. By the stirring up of dust and sand, the negative ions are removed. A positive to negative ratio of 35 to 1 is often reached by the Chinook wind that plagues the Rockies and the Southern California desert of Santa Ana. They are the ill winds that blow no good.

On the seashore where the surf is creating spray, the ratio is 2 to 1 on the negative side. This is restorative and energizing for us.

SPECIAL BENEFITS OF A SHOWER. Taking a shower is invigorating for all the reasons that you think, plus one more: The falling water creates thousands of negative ions by splitting neutral particles of air and freeing the ions. You benefit in many ways by the extra negative ions. You are probably not consciously aware of the specifics, and even if you were, you would never dream of attributing them to the shower you just took.

IMPROVED OXYGEN DELIVERY. Most researchers believe that negative ions improve our capacity to absorb and utilize oxygen. They accelerate the delivery of life-sustaining oxygen to our cells and tissues.

Other specific health benefits of increased negative ions in the air you breathe, while taking a shower and for a while thereafter, have been researched in Europe. They include a reduction of anxiety. This is traced to an increase in brain alpha-wave output, which has an overall calming effect.

These benefits also include a heightening of appetite, increased thirst and stimulated sexual behavior.

Calm, hungry, loving—sounds like the Hawaiians!

There are a number of air ionizers on the market. Many are priced at under $100. Examples are the Omega 700 Ionizer by Bio/Environmental Systems, Inc., 121 S. Hartz Ave., Danville, California 94526, Air Energizer by Ion Research Center, Box 6440, Boulder Creek, California 95006, and the Hybrid 402 by Quantum Instrument Co., 3515 N. 25th Pl., Phoenix, Arizona 85016. Check your phone book's yellow pages. We cannot bring clean Hawaiian air to you, but this is one way you can come a step closer to breathing pure air in your home.

FRESH DRINKING WATER—
ITS IMPORTANCE TO YOUR HEALTH

Too bad it isn't as easy to create country-fresh water as it is to provide country-fresh air through ionizing. But there is one advantage in the case of water.

You breathe air wherever you go. So there are air ionizers for the car, for suites of offices and for the home. But you usually drink water in only one or two places.

If there could be sources of fresh, unchemicalized water available to you, you would be privy to another Hawaiian and Polynesian health secret.

Our water is not fluoridated. It is not even chlorinated, unless you are in a hotel or restaurant. There are few water systems in the United States that can make this claim.

PURER WATER. In late 1975, health-minded people breathed a sigh of relief when the Safe Drinking Water Act was adopted, which said in part, "No national primary drinking water regulation may require the addition of any substance for preventive health-care purposes unrelated to contamination of drinking water.'' It seemed that at last the battle against fluorine and its known dangers was won.

Not so. The Environmental Protection Agency was quick to point out that the law did not bar states and municipalities from introducing fluorine into their water systems.

So, you still need to search for pure water.

SPRING WATER. One answer is bottled spring water. Most business areas are supplied with this service for their water coolers.

DISTILLED WATER. Another source is distilled water. This is available in many supermarkets. Since pharmacists are required to use distilled water in making prescriptions, all pharmacists have a source and if they do not actually sell distilled water, they can direct you to where you can buy it.

The taste of distilled water is flat and "empty." A few drops of lemon will help.

Hawaiian water is full of minerals. Distilled water is not. Bottled spring water comes closest to duplicating the water here.

However, so many people drink bottled soda or beer instead of water that these products present a greater problem than does the local water supply.

OTHER DRINKS—AND WHAT TO AVOID

Starting with bottled soda, the worst ones for you are the colas. Besides sugar, they also contain caffeine. Next in harmfulness come all of the other sweet flavors, which still contain plenty of sugar that creates toxins in the body. Even the low-calorie soft drink can be hard on you, as there is increasing evidence that the synthetic sweeteners are not as innocent as their low-calorie profile would have you believe. Some have already been barred from use. Others may follow.

NEUTRAL SOFT DRINKS. Sparkling water and mineral water offer the least objectionable factors, if you must drink soda. You can add lemon, vanilla or other flavoring. Waiters who once judged the sophistication of their patrons by the wine they ordered, now do so by the bottled water they order. There are highly carbonated waters, medium carbonated waters and flat waters. They clear the palate between courses of a meal and also provide a refreshing break in the afternoon or evening. The current best seller in the country is Perrier, somewhat on the higher carbonation level. At the lighter carbonation level is Forrarelle.

A BETTER BEER. As for beers, they are all made with water from municipal water supplies. Primo, a beer bottled in Hawai'i since 1897, used to be the only exception, but as we write this, the Primo facilities in Honolulu are being closed by the parent company, Schlitz, and by the time you read this, Primo will be being bottled on the mainland. The present label on the bottle will have to be changed, but it now reads:

> *Pure Hawaiian water, naturally filtered through thousands of layers of lava rock, is combined with the finest quality brewery ingredients to give Primo beer a distinctive light golden taste.*

Although we've lost a beer brewery, Honolulu now boasts the first *sake* brewery outside Japan. *Sake* (pronounced "sah-kay") has been brewed from rice for over 1600 years. The predominantly Japanese population has made Hawai'i a big market for *sake*.

ALCOHOLIC PROTEIN. Recently, *sake* has been found to contain essential amino acids so that it can contribute to protein in the body, instead of the fat and carbohydrates that are present in most liquors.

Here in Hawai'i, most people drink *sake* warmed in a porcelain container and served in little porcelain cups. But colorless *sake* tastes good warmed or not, in a cup or a shot glass.

If we were asked to name three beverages besides water that were health secrets in Hawai'i, we would certainly name Primo Beer, *sake,* and . . .

THE FROSTY DELIGHT THAT HAWAIIANS ENJOY

Have you ever heard of "shave ice"? It is pidgin English for "shaved ice," the ice cream cone of Hawai'i.

LOW-CALORIE THIRST QUENCHER. This type of "ice cream" has it all over the standard cone in the health department. Besides satisfying thirst, while an ice cream cone creates thirst, shave ice has fewer calories and less sugar. Anything with less sugar has got to contribute to a longer life.

What is shave ice? It is ice that has been crushed into a snowy mush.

It is then piled high on a cup and munched like a cone. Many enjoy it plain, but you can have a squirt of flavored syrup on it.

We have yet to see ice cream vending trucks in Hawai'i, like the familiar Good Humor man on the mainland. But anyone who has $250 to invest in a shave ice machine can go into business in Hawai'i, and there are a number of shave ice outlets all over the islands.

You might start a new health practice on the mainland. It won't have the advantage of pure Hawaiian water, but your product will be more refreshing than ice cream. Here are two sources to write to about a shave ice machine:

- Hotei-Ya, Ala Moana Shopping Center, 1450 Ala Moana Blvd., Honolulu, Hawaii 96814, for the more economical type.
- Job Popcorn, 1816 Hart St., Honolulu, Hawaii 96819, for the professional type.

Years ago, a block of ice was planed to get a cupful of the frosty stuff. Later came a cranked model that rotated a blade under the ice. Today, the professional machine uses an electrically driven turntable with the block of ice held in a four-pronged vise-like gadget which presses the ice onto a whirling blade. This "snow plow" creates a cool, clear icy powder.

You can come close to this product if you have a juicer. Many juicers come with an ice crusher attachment. This makes a reasonable facsimile of shave ice. Be sure to thaw the ice a bit. When it's good and wet it sticks together better and holds the syrup well.

The really health-minded folks use no syrup. Diabetics also avoid the syrup. But those who want a little more taste to their shave ice ask for one of the many flavored syrups that are available. The number one favorite in Hawai'i is strawberry. Just a squirt goes a long way. Yes, it does contain sugar, but not that much compared with sherbet or ice cream.

TEN MORE TIPS TO COMBAT AIR AND WATER POLLUTION

Pure air and pure water are Hawai'i's heritage. All of Polynesia is similarly blessed. Of what benefit is it to mainlanders to know that these two factors make a sizable contribution to longevity, when most mainland air and most mainland water are polluted and chemicalized?

Our chief contribution here has been to remind you about ionizers to improve the quality of your air and to look to bottled spring water to improve the quality of your drinking water.

The problem is insidious because it erodes health so slowly. One more day of impure air or impure water will make so little difference that we let the days go by until it is too late. It's just like the cigarette smoker who is told by his doctor that each cigarette takes five minutes off his total life expectancy. He still lights up for five minutes of "pleasure" now in exchange for five minutes of oblivion later.

Most people in Hawai'i and Polynesia take fresh air and fresh water for granted. Unfortunately, you cannot take your air and your water for granted. You need to be aware of the air you are breathing and the water you are drinking.

Scientists and health professionals, recognizing the problem, have published a number of combative measures that anyone can take when forced to live in an urban environment and drink chemicalized water. Here are some of the most practical tips.

AIR

1. *FRESH AIR HOLIDAYS*. Take holidays in the country. Drive out of the city some weekend or even just for an evening. A two-week vacation in the mountains or at the seashore is especially beneficial. Any time spent in pure air gives your lungs, liver and other vital organs a chance to recuperate, to regenerate and to build up a resistance to the next dose of toxins.

2. *AIR PURIFYING PLANTS*. Keep growing plants in your home and in window boxes. They help to purify the air. Besides decorative plants, grow herbs or plants that provide food.

3. *TOXIN PREVENTIVE DETOURS*. Drive on the less traveled side streets to avoid being tied up in traffic and its carbon monoxide clouds. Breathe shallow breaths when you're exposed to exhaust or smokers' fumes; breath deeply as you emerge into fresher air.

WATER

4. Avoid drinking restaurant water. Postpone your drink until you return home to your own purer water.

5. *SOFTENED WATER*. Consider using a water-softener attachment in your home if the municipal supply is hard water (over-mineralized).

TOTAL ENVIRONMENT

6. *WASHED FOOD*. Wash supermarket fruits and vegetables with warm water and soap. Rinsing alone does not get rid of poison sprays. Peel fruits and vegetables that cannot be washed.

7. Favor organically grown fruits and vegetables that have not been sprayed. You can buy these at your health food store or grow your own.

8. Stop using chemical toxins in your own home, like aerosol sprays, so-called air fresheners, cleaning fluids, detergents and insect repellents.

9. When clothing is returned from the dry cleaner, air it out before you wear it.

10. Fortify your system, so that it can better handle air and water pollutants, by eating a natural diet that is high in vitamins and minerals and by taking a wide range of vitamin and mineral supplements.

GETTING THE MOST REST FROM SLEEP

Fresh air, fresh water and plenty of sleep are three basic elements of a healthier life.

People who have heard the old maxim, "Early to bed and early to rise makes one healthy, wealthy and wise," do not seem to pay much attention to it. On the other hand, in Hawai'i, where we have never heard that advice, people go to bed early and get up early as part of their natural life style.

The standard 9 to 5 hours on the mainland are far from standard in Hawai'i. Many offices open at 7:00 a.m. If any hour is to be called standard, 8:00 a.m. would be more like it. Rare is the office that waits until 9:00 a.m. to open. Even banks open at 8:30.

Home-bound traffic begins at 3:30 p.m. The mainland 5:00 rush is on at 4:00 in Honolulu. By 8:00 or 9:00 in the evening, the streets are quite deserted.

This is not the case in Waikiki or other visitor destinations. Drive along Kalakaua Avenue in the heart of Waikiki even after midnight and you will find the sidewalks alive with people. But drive along that same avenue at its other extremity in a local residential and business area and all will be quiet and dark.

People in Honolulu hesitate to telephone their friends or relatives after 9:00 p.m.—they might be asleep. While you may listen to the 11:00 news on the mainland, we tune in to the late news at 9:30 p.m. By 10:00, most people in the city are on their way to bed—we are!—and in the country they are probably fast asleep by that time.

Of course, there is no scientific proof that the early-to-bed maxim has any validity. But by and large, Hawaiians are early to bed, early to rise people. And since Hawaiians are a healthy people, we must look at this practice at least as circumstantial evidence that "early to bed and early to rise" contributes to total health.

THE BEST SLEEP. There is one persistent claim, that also has not been proved, that sleep obtained before midnight is the most valuable sleep. This falls into the same mystical category as the claim that your head should be pointed north while sleeping, for maximum benefit. With all the research going on today in the field of psychotronics, electromagnetic effects and the nature of life energy, we might very well come up with some findings that throw some credibility on such presently little understood factors that affect sleep.

Meanwhile, we vote for "early to bed." We will leave "early to rise" to your discretion. Many people spend some time awake in bed, either right after retiring or later on during the night. We have no advice on the total hours of sleep you need for optimum benefit. There seems to be no characteristic that is peculiar to Hawai'i and Polynesia. People here, on the average, get seven to nine hours of sleep a night, pretty much the same as mainland averages.

As for helping you to fall asleep, we do have one Hawaiian and Polynesian secret.

NATURAL "SLEEPING PILL." The dried leaves and stems of passionflower calm hyperactive people and induce natural sleep, with no disturbance of normal cerebral functions. There is no known toxicity to passionflower when used in small doses. A half teaspoonful, brewed as a tea in a cup of water, will induce sleep as effectively as drugstore products and with none of the side effects.

Passionflower *(Passiflora incarnata)* is becoming more well-known and more widely used around the world. It is used in Italy to quiet hyperactive children. According to ethnobiologist Michael Weiner of the University of California, passionflower may be an alternative to presently used tranquilizers.

Because it is now recognized as a homeopathic remedy for insomnia, it can be obtained through homeopathic medicine practitioners or by writing Standard Homeopathic Company, P.O. Box 6106, Los Angeles, California 90061.

NIGHT AIR. Night air is fresher than daytime air. Open your windows more, weather permitting, and get plenty of fresh air while you're sleeping.

We were mainland city folks once. We know the tendency to sleep with the windows open "just a crack." Now we know that it is better to have an extra blanket and sleep with fresher air. Try it. Notice the difference in the way you feel when you arise in the morning.

8

Deriving Health Benefits from Sun and Sea

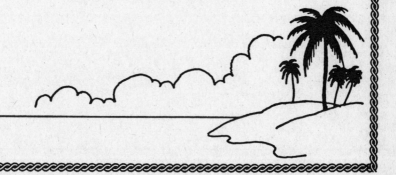

Even though it is made up of islands, the 50th state has less shoreline than a number of our other states. Yet, the people who live in Hawai'i appreciate their shoreline. The beaches belong to the people and, even though private homes may front the beach, public rights of way give easy beach access to all.

In this chapter, we examine just how health benefits are derived from the sun and the sea, as well as some health dangers. In the process, we discover:

A POSSIBLE CURE FOR BALDNESS

PREVENTING SKIN CANCER

PREVENTING SKIN AGING

PREVENTING WRINKLES

A PLANT SUNBURN RELIEVER

A FRUIT SUNBURN RELIEVER

AVOIDING HARMFUL SUN

ANTI-AGING VITAMIN

SUN-RESISTING SUPPLE-MENTS

FRESH AIR BENEFITS

DARING ACTIVITIES

PASSIVE ACTIVITIES

ESCAPING STRESS

SAND WALKING THERAPY

MINERAL BATH THERAPY

SWIMMING FOR HEALTH

WATER CALISTHENICS

A NEW WATER SPORT

RUNNING FOR YOUR HEART

SWIMMING FOR YOUR HEART

BETTER CIRCULATION

BETTER COORDINATION

BUSTLINE IMPROVEMENT

WEIGHT CONTROL

The sun and the beaches of Hawai'i make a solid contribution to the health of the people who live there. The sun and the beaches do not make this contribution by their mere presence. They have to be used. And it is the use each person makes of them that contributes to his or her health.

In this chapter, we are going to examine these uses. You have sunshine where you live, perhaps not as bright as the Hawaiian sun, but nevertheless you can get the tanning effects of the sun's rays. You have bodies of water within reasonable driving distance—perhaps a lake, pond, river, ocean or even just a swimming pool.

So you can look at Hawaiian practices and adapt them for your local situation—for the betterment of your health.

Few Hawaiians are sun worshippers. You do not see people here on roofs and balconies or in parks, stripped to the waist or in shorts and halters, as you might see in New York or Chicago, getting their share of the sun.

Here they prefer the shade of a palm tree because the sun is so strong that just getting from place to place or engaging in some sport, such as jogging, provides enough sun.

The average resident of Honolulu probably gets as much sun every day just going about his or her daily routine as does the New Yorker who spends an hour at Jones Beach each day during July and August, except that the Honolulu person has it all year round.

Even in their religious background, the Hawaiians did not worship the sun. There is some epigraphical evidence that the early Polynesians may have come from Egypt. The Egyptians did worship the sun. Their sun god was named Ra, and he sailed the heavens in a boat. The Greeks saw the sun as their god Apollo, and also as Helios, who drove his burning chariot across the sky. The Aztecs of Mexico considered themselves as descendants of the sun, as did the Hopi Indians. The Emperor of Japan is still looked on by the Japanese as being a descendant of the sun.

THE SUN'S DUAL ROLE IN YOUR LIFE

The sun keeps this planet from being a cold, dark, lifeless orb. Plant and animal life depend on the sun for their very existence.

Yet, just what specific benefits are derived from the direct rays of the sun is still an unsolved problem. Back in 1903, a Danish scientist won the

Nobel Prize for discovering that skin tuberculosis can be cured with the sun's rays.

It was about that same time that Paul Bragg was dying of tuberculosis in an Adirondacks sanitarium at the age of 16. Here, the prescribed treatment was indoor bed rest. His nurse convinced his parents that he should travel to her country, Switzerland, where they knew how to treat tuberculosis. There Paul Bragg recovered rapidly. The cure consisted of plenty of outdoor sunshine and activity, including nude baths in the snow.

We know a little bit more today about the sun's benefits, but not much more. We know, for instance, that a child's body needs at least a few minutes a day of the direct rays of the sun in order to metabolize vitamin D. Once the bones have fully matured, this need no longer exists.

The ultraviolet rays of the sun have been associated with physical fitness. These rays have also been found to be therapeutic for such skin diseases as eczema, acne and psoriasis.

Full spectrum light from the sun, not necessarily direct, has been found by researchers to have important effects. Male rats bred in artificial light became irritable and developed cannibalistic tendencies, whereas full spectrum natural light made them docile and gentle.

Dr. John N. Ott, in his book *Health and Light,** brings up example after example of the vital necessity of full spectrum light. Mink breeders found poor quality in the fur of minks that were kept away from sunlight, while those in full spectrum sunlight developed luxuriant fur, leading us to wonder if baldness is not caused by a sun deficiency.

A POSSIBLE CURE FOR BALDNESS. Although we know of no study of this factor made in Hawai'i, just looking around gives one the impression that baldness is a mainland import. Rare is the native Hawaiian who is bald. If you see a bald person, he is most likely a recent arrival. At visitor destinations like Waikiki, you see plenty of bald heads.

Other benefits derived from the sun are presently being researched, such as the effect of full spectrum light, as opposed to window light from which certain ranges of the sun's rays have been screened out, on the pineal and pituitary glands, and via these glands on general health. Therein may be a sun-drenched Hawaiian and Polynesian health secret still to be revealed.

---

*Devin-Adair Co., Old Greenwich, Connecticut, 1974.

We seem to know more about the dangers of the sun than we do about its benefits.

According to the American Cancer Society, some 115,000 new skin cancers are detected each year in the United States and, of these, 5000 will be fatal.

The sun is the cause. It puts out more dangerous radiation than our bodies can take. The visible rays range from 2500 to 4000 angstroms in wavelength, an angstrom being one hundred-millionth of a centimeter. The ultraviolet rays range from 2900 to 3200 angstroms. These are the cancer-producing wavelengths. They are also the tanning and burning wavelengths.

It is a quirk of human nature that light-skinned people seek to be suntanned, while people with dark skin prefer to remain as light as they can be. It is a quirk of mother nature that light-skinned people who consider a suntan to be the "in" thing are the ones who can tolerate sun the least.

PREVENTING SKIN CANCER. You can prevent skin cancer caused by the sun by measuring your time in the sun, as you would measure your time under a sun lamp.

PREVENTING SKIN AGING AND WRINKLES. In the process, you will also be minimizing other unwanted effects of the sun: leathery skin, aging and wrinkles.

If you would like to see the effects that the sun has had on your skin over the years, compare the skin on your face with the skin on your buttocks. Unless you are a full-time nudist, there should be quite a difference.

HOW TO GET THE SUN'S BENEFITS
WITHOUT ITS HARM

We are forever seeing white-skinned arrivals sunning on the beach at Waikiki and turning slightly pink. This can happen to unconditioned skin in about 30 minutes midday in Hawai'i, all year round.

"Pardon us, Sir (or Miss)," we venture, "but you had better protect your skin."

"Thanks. I'll be OK."

Coming up—one ruined vacation. The tropical sun of Hawai'i burns faster than the color of the skin can respond, meaning that even back in the hotel room the burn will continue to redden and worsen.

A PLANT SUNBURN RELIEVER; A FRUIT SUNBURN RELIEVER. Here are two reminders of natural healing agents for sunburn. We have mentioned *aloe*. The sap from a leaf of this plant squeezed onto your finger and then spread on the affected skin can bring immediate relief. If you have access to papayas, mash the whole fruit, skin and all, in your blender and apply the paste.

The best approach, though, is prevention.

Mad dogs and Englishmen, said Noel Coward, go out in the midday sun. We do not appear to have very many of either in Hawai'i. People tend to stay in the shade. If they must be exposed to the sun, they take precautions. The men wear sun visors and the women carry parasols.

Once the sun is well past its zenith and there is more atmosphere cutting down on the ultraviolet rays, the danger of overexposure diminishes. Hawaiians seem to know this instinctively. By midafternoon, the beaches are more crowded and games more visible.

The lesson for mainlanders is to get plenty of sun but not too much sun. In the northern states, it is more difficult to get plenty than it is to get too much. Winter cold prevents exposure of more than the face, and summers are short. Still, overexposure is possible in Wisconsin, Washington and Maine during May, June, July and August.

Three factors affect the strength of the sun: proximity to the equator, proximity to June 21 (in the northern hemisphere), and proximity to noon.

AVOIDING HARMFUL SUN. Note that in some southern extremities of the United States the sun crosses its zenith just before and just after June 21, making a few weeks at that time of the year an extended period of maximum sun.

These maximum periods are danger periods. Exposure to the sun should be rationed carefully at these times. Precautions should be taken against the ultraviolet rays, and we will mention the best of these in a moment.

A few weeks away from seasonal zenith and an hour or two away from daily zenith take the "sting" away. Then the sun becomes your friend, not your enemy.

Sensitive skin can burn even in the shade and even under water. The sun can penetrate water and is also reflected by white sand. Count all time spent out of doors as time in the sun.

SUNTAN LOTIONS, SUNTAN OILS AND SUN SCREENS

The suntan oil of the Pacific is coconut oil. It is available commercially wherever suntan lotions and oils are sold. Although extracted with petroleum solvents from the dried meat, it is a pure, natural product. Coconut oil keeps the tan even and the skin soft. It does not protect skin from ultraviolet rays.

Cocoa butter has nothing to do with the coconut. It is a byproduct of the manufacture of chocolate and is available in pharmacies. It, too, is an excellent sun lotion in that it provides an even tan and keeps the skin lubricated.

Coconut butter has plenty to do with the coconut. It is made from coconut milk just the way ordinary butter is made from ordinary milk. First the coconut milk is allowed to stand so that the cream can rise. The cream is skimmed off the top and then churned until it becomes a thick butter. Coconut butter is not only a delicious, healthful food—perhaps the most wholesome of all fats—it is also the natural cosmetic of the South Pacific.

It is used both by the lovely maidens and by the rugged fishermen who need to protect their skin from the salty spray.

However, coconut butter is not available commercially even on the islands. It is made by those who have access to coconuts and who value it as a cosmetic and sun lotion.

Since this is a health book, we are less interested in an even tan than we are in adequate sun protection for your skin. Suntan oils and lotions do not protect you. Only sun screens protect you. A sun screen is a substance that prevents ultraviolet rays from penetrating it.

A chemical has been found that screens out the cancer-causing rays of the sun. It is called para-aminobenzoic acid (PABA).

PREVENTING SKIN CANCER. Norman Goldstein, M.D.,* a Honolulu dermatologist, recently tested PABA under controlled conditions to confirm its protection against skin cancer. Two groups of mice were exposed to the sun. One group was covered with PABA; the other was not. The mice that were not protected developed 15 times as many tumors.

---

*The Skin You Live In, Hart Publishing Co., Inc., New York, 1978.

Make sure that the product you buy includes the ingredient PABA. The label can also read "para-aminobenzoic acid" or "p-aminobenzoic acid." It comes with an oil, cream or alcohol base. Dr. Goldstein prefers the alcohol base because it penetrates the skin better and gives greater protection. One example is Presun. Others are Pabafilm, Maxafilm and Solbar.

When you walk into your pharmacy, you will not see these products displayed as prominently as such nationally promoted lotions as Tanya and Coppertone. But despite what the ads say, these latter types of suntan oils and lotions offer no real protection from skin cancer. Moisturizing oils, lotions, butters, cosmetic stainers and bronzers offer no protection against the sun's harmful rays. Only sun screens do—like PABA.

Some persons are sensitive to sun screens. If one you are using causes irritation, discontinue its use. If the irritation persists, see your dermatologist.

Most sun worshippers find a convenient answer in PABA. It can be put on early in the day and it lasts, resisting perspiration. It even improves with time. However, if you are in the sun for as long as three hours, or if you take a swim, a second application is recommended.

Enjoy your tan, and enjoy healthy skin.

BEAUTY TIPS FOR SUNNERS

We who live in the sun learn more about its aging effects and how to prevent them. We know the effects of sea and salt on the skin and hair and how to minimize them. Since women are more sensitive to these effects, the next few paragraphs are directed mainly to them.

When you are in the sun, you perspire to cause evaporation which cools the body, thus keeping the sun-exposed body at an even temperature. When you perspire, you lose minerals and water-soluble vitamins.

Something else happens. The skin thickens to increase its protection, decreasing pore effectiveness and reducing the skin's elimination capability. This puts more of the load on the kidneys and lungs. In addition, melamine, the skin pigmentation that gives you color, requires B vitamins in its production, further depleting the body of that essential.

You can build up a resistance to these effects through a program of nutrition that includes the right vitamins and minerals.

ANTI-AGING VITAMIN. Vitamin E is good insurance against wrinkles. It is gaining a reputation for being an anti-aging vitamin.

Sidney Petrie, noted nutrition expert, in his book *The Wonder Protein Diet,** states, "The only thing holding back an explosion of professional enthusiasm for the life-prolonging properties of vitamin E is the scientific understanding of *how* it works. There is no doubt *that* it works."

Petrie cites laboratory work by gerontologists that points to a five- to ten-year lengthening of life span through the use of vitamin E.

Its effects are therefore not merely cosmetic. Your skin remains youthful, despite exposure to the sun, because it *is* youthful.

SUN-RESISTING SUPPLEMENTS. B vitamins are another good supplement to take. They build up your hair's resistance to sun and surf. Throw in some vitamin C for general resistance. The supplement RNA, another substance with a suspected longevity factor, increases the skin's moisture level.

We will leave the external care of your hair and skin to you, as you know your particular conditions. Just remember the wearing effects of the sun while you enjoy its "healthing" effects.

THE BEACH—TO GO OR NOT TO GO

Tom H. hates the beach. When he lived on the mainland, he avoided the beach. He believes that anyone over 25 who gets into a pair of swimming trunks or a bikini is an embarrassment to family and friends. He does not like the sand. It gets into all the wrong places, such as in your hair and inside your suit. He claims that men are left with an itchy feeling no matter how long they shower, because they still have sand hiding in sensitive areas. He hates to be a prisoner to beach towel or mat. ("You're afraid to leave it for fear that someone will rip off your personal belongings.") And he prefers not to be surrounded by "half-naked strangers, screeching children, caterwauling transistor radios and ravishing creatures in revealing bikinis who make you feel old and fat."

Nevertheless, Tom goes down to the seashore. He has fun. He escapes the stress of the Honolulu business world. He gets fresh air, sun

---

*Parker Publishing Company, Inc., West Nyack, New York, 1979.

and exercise. His favorite seashore area, now that he lives in Hawai'i, is Kona on the Big Island. Why? Because there's no sand.

Kona's shoreline is rocky, but there is plenty of fun to be had at the seashore without a beach. If you live near water, but not near a beach, you may be able to borrow some activity ideas from Kona.

FRESH AIR BENEFITS. Keep in mind that going to the ocean's edge is good for you. Going to a river, lake, bay or stream is good for you. Salt air, ionized air, outdoor air, fresher air is good for you.

What do you do when you get there?

In Kona, the fishing is great. Beaches, especially crowded beaches, tend to interfere with fishing. There is sport fishing, where you hire a boat and go after the big marlin. But there is also lots of shore fishing. Kids, from 8 to 80, fish successfully off the rocks with nets or poles.

The fresh air is good for you and, when coupled with the fresh fish, you score two points for health!

In Kona there are motorboating, sailboating and sightseeing cruises. There is outrigger canoe paddling. We doubt whether you will ever see an outrigger canoe in your local mainland waters, but then you have rowboats, which are just as rare here and just as good for exercise and fun.

You do not need sand to snorkel or scuba dive, and the equipment is not that expensive. Exploring the underwater areas may not be as dramatic where you live as it is in Kona, where dazzling undersea coral and rock formations attract rainbows of fish. But wherever you dive, it is still good fun and good exercise.

DARING ACTIVITIES. There are waves for surfing in Kona. And there is water skiing. These activities are for the braver souls. And for the still braver souls, there is para-sailing, where you are hitched to a large kite, pulled by a motorboat and lift off, sailing through the sky perhaps 100 feet up. Or, you might try balloon jib sailing, where you are yanked off the boat deck by the ballooning sail and held swinging in the air for as long as your courage holds out.

These are relatively safe, yet invigorating and exhilarating experiences. You forget your stressful problems. You return home feeling physically and spiritually "high," as if the universe had given you a massage.

We do speak from experience. The experience of others! We have never tried these daring sports.

PASSIVE ACTIVITIES. We tend to be boat watchers, dry-land surfers

("Why didn't he grab that wave; it was perfect!"), and courage admirers.

We get healthy by watching. We get appropriate amounts of sun. We get fresh air. We walk, sit and swim. We have fun.

These are the important health factors. You do not have to dangle 100 feet in the air and be that much closer to the sun to get your sunshine requirements. You do not have to "wipe out" and be thrown about in the breakers with your surfboard to get invigorating exercise. And your lungs can take in no more fresh air under a billowing sail than they can take in on the beach.

All of which says, "Go!"

ESCAPING STRESS. No matter what you like or dislike about what others are doing at the shore or on the beach, go and "do your own thing."

It takes you out of the stress of civilized life and into the stress-less therapy of nature.

A HEALTHFUL ASPECT OF BEACH SAND

If you live on the mainland and come to Hawai'i, your feet will feel the difference in the sand.

Mainland beaches have sand that is made up largely of quartz crystals. It is soft and powdery.

Hawaiian white sand is made from shell and coral fragments. Hawaiian black sand is pulverized lava. Both sands are hard and firm compared to East Coast and West Coast sand beaches.

We came to Hawai'i from Long Island, New York. There the sand is as soft as anywhere in the world. We were a bit disappointed in the Waikiki sand until we learned that walking on hard sand is a very special therapy.

The old Hawaiians knew about something that has only recently been rediscovered—foot reflexology. Inside the soles of the feet are nerve endings that go to all parts of the body. By massaging a certain zone of the foot, you can increase the circulation to a particular ailing part of the body.

SAND WALKING THERAPY. The *kahunas* advised long walks in bare feet on the hard sand. This was tantamount to a massage for the soles of the feet and, via the nerve endings, to the ailing organ or area of the body.

L. L. Schneider, D.C., N.D., in his book *Old Fashioned Health Remedies That Work Best,** talks about the old way of walking on gravel as a similar "massage." Apparently, the Hawaiians were not alone in their understanding of the importance of the soles of the feet.

We now have a greater respect for the harder sand of Hawai'i. We take daily walks on it. You can see many other people doing likewise, some making it a daily ritual to walk several miles in bare feet on the sand.

Wally S., an escapee from California's space industries—where stress was a constant threat—walks three miles daily, stopping along the way to talk to friends. He is now a healthy-looking specimen as he pushes 60.

If the sand is soft where you go to the beach, walk along the water's edge. Here the wetness compacts the sand and makes it exactly what the *kahuna* ordered.

If you have no sand, use grandad's method of gravel walking. Or, if this is not convenient for you city dwellers, roll a golf ball around on the floor with your bare feet pressing down on it. Any commercial foot massaging device is also good, such as the "Footsie Roller."**

WHAT THE OCEAN CAN MEAN TO YOUR HEALTH

Mineral baths have been recognized by man for centuries as having curative effects.

MINERAL BATH THERAPY. In Europe, especially Germany and Russia, there are uncountable mineral spas where millions of people go annually. Modern scientists have studied these baths and conclude that they do indeed work. Many are now under the direction of licensed medical doctors. Their patients are helped in the relief of just about every medical difficulty, including nervous disorders, arthritis, heart disease, circulatory problems and even senility.

There are mineral baths in the United States, in places such as Saratoga, New York; White Sulphur Springs, West Virginia; and numerous places in the West. But the water that has the greatest curative

---

*Parker Publishing Company, Inc., West Nyack, New York, 1977.
**Available from Natural Energies, Box 350, Whitmore Lake, Michigan 48189.

powers—according to one of the world's foremost nutritionists and naturopathic physicians, Paavo O. Airola, Ph.D., N.D.—is the salt water of the ocean.

Dr. Airola notes that minerals in the ocean are absorbed through the skin during ocean bathing and even by inhaling the mineral-rich air of the seashore. For those who cannot avail themselves of this therapy because of inland locations, he recommends making your own salt water bath by dissolving three or four pounds of sea salt in a half-filled bathtub of cool water. Rub or brush yourself briskly while in the tub and then dry yourself vigorously. If sea salt is not available in your health food store, make your own with one part Epsom salt, one part magnesium chloride and seven parts common table salt.

Of course, the homemade mineral bath deprives you of the benefits of swimming.

There are probably more annual man-woman-child-hours of swimming enjoyed in Hawai'i, proportionate to its population, than in any other state in the Union. Every day is a swimmable day in Hawai'i, considering the water and air temperatures which change very little.

SWIMMING FOR HEALTH. Perhaps it is only based on circumstantial evidence to say that, because the longest living people swim the most, swimming is good for you. But swimming has long been recognized as one of the most beneficial exercises for the human body. Until recently, it was recommended as physical therapy even more than running.

In Hawai'i, there are annual distance swims in which everyone takes part—male and female, young and old. A two- to three-mile swim in the open ocean ends on the Waikiki Beach, where tourists are impressed as they watch young men, old men, girls and matrons arrive at the finish line in the best of condition and spirits.

Another Hawaiian event, the annual Honolulu Triatholon, combines a rough-water swim followed by an island bicycle race around O'ahu (about 75 miles), followed by a 26-mile marathon. Would you agree that people who live in Hawai'i love the outdoors?

But swimming even for just a few minutes improves the circulation. The water massages the body. The muscles, emphasizing movement rather than tension, receive a physical treat. Calories are burned away and the figure improves. Tissues are toned. You feel like a new person.

EXERCISING IN THE WATER

Swimming is not the only exercise that you can enjoy in the ocean, lake or pool. The ocean claims an exclusive when it comes to body surfing—getting a ride in on the waves without a surfboard. But lakes and pools have their advantages, too.

Quiet water gives you the opportunity to use flotation devices to enjoy the tranquil effects of being away from the "action." Rubber rafts, mattresses and life preservers give you a chance to relax on nature's water bed.

WATER CALISTHENICS. Quiet water gives you a chance to do underwater calisthenics. These have now become quite popular in Hawai'i and on the mainland, in municipal pools, as well as YMCA and YWCA facilities.

Here are a few examples. They are done standing waist deep to chest deep in the water.

Aqua-Jog

Jog in place. First move the feet up and down. Then add a movement forward, still standing in the same place. Now thrust the jogging feet slightly backward. Now to the right. Now to the left.

Cossack

Start with arms horizontal or even with the water surface in front of you. Now as you press the water down sharply with both arms, jump up, kicking your feet out and forward in Cossack dance fashion. Repeat 12 times.

Arm Circles

With shoulders almost even with the surface of the water, extend both arms out well under the water. Now make circles with the arms as you begin to jog. Rotate the arms forward. Then repeat the exercise rotating the arms backward.

A NEW ACTIVITY FOR THE SKILLFUL

One day in mid-1978, we saw a strange sight. A man was riding a surfboard with a sail on it. "How unique!" we thought. "He must be an acrobat to stay on." And off he went.

A NEW WATER SPORT. Now, one year later, Hawai'i is the mecca of wind surfing, a craze that is sweeping the world. According to those in the know, Hawai'i produces the best custom boards, the fastest sails and the top wind surfers. A 15-year-old O'ahu lad has won the world wind surfing championship for the third straight time, the most recent contest having been held at Cancun, Mexico on the Yucatan Peninsula. Before that, it was at the Bahamas and then at Sardinia off the coast of Italy.

Wind surfing requires strength and coordination. It is usually taught on the beach with a mock-up of the real thing: a surfboard with a sail, mounted on a rotating stand. All the mechanics of the sport can be learned on dry land. Most people learn the basics in a single half-hour lesson using this simulator.

Then come the health benefits, and we hear raves in this department. A former athlete suffering from chronic backache took up wind surfing and, within three weeks of daily trips, he was free of his problem and able to rejoin his team.

A young woman suffering prematurely with arthritis in her hands and ankle joints got permanent relief after a few days of wind surfing.

One day this special sport will be analyzed by therapists to see what is at work to make it not only fun but also powerful medicine for the body. Meanwhile, more and more people in Hawai'i are taking up wind surfing seriously, and benefiting from it. No doubt you will be hearing about wind surfing in your part of the country soon.

RUNNING VERSUS SWIMMING AS A HEALTH PRACTICE

Running is as much of a craze in Hawai'i as anywhere else in the United States. However, we cannot point to running as a Hawaiian and Polynesian health secret. When we first came here as visitors in the early 1960s, a runner was somebody trying to catch a bus. Today, runners and joggers are everywhere you look—in the parks, on the highways, along sidewalks, even in the downtown business district.

Running or jogging is a Johnny-come-lately to the Hawaiian health scene, perhaps too lately to have affected the longevity statistics.

Honolulu has now had its sixth annual marathon. Over 10,000 runners participated in the December 1979 event which covered 26.2 miles. No records were set because Hawai'i's temperatures in the 70s and 80s are far from the ideal running temperature of the low 50s, and its 50 to 60 humidity is far above the ideal running humidity of 20.

RUNNING FOR YOUR HEART. Although over 2000 of the entries came from the mainland and as far away as Japan, Germany, Singapore and Australia, many participants were members of an ongoing Honolulu Marathon Clinic, a physical fitness activity directed by a physician named Dr. Jack H. Scaff, Jr. Participation in the clinic's running activities is a prescription for many heart patients on the island.

But there is another clinic being formed—a Swimming Stroke Clinic. Directing this water route is Jan Prins, swimming coach and pool director at the University of Hawaii. He advocates swimming as both rehabilitative and preventive medicine.

SWIMMING FOR YOUR HEART. Swimming is a natural alternative to running. Some people just do not like to run. Perhaps they have bad feet or a bothersome back. Quoting the clinic's brochure, "Our clinic is designed for all persons interested in using swimming as an alternative form of developing cardiovascular fitness. Running is an excellent form of exercise, but it is often accompanied by soreness in the joints and lower back. Swimming, being a non-weightbearing form of exercise, eliminates these possible complications."

Personally, we favor swimming. Somehow, running on hard pavements, such as sidewalks and streets, seems unnatural and a possible strain on internal systems. Swimming is a more gentle exercise. And it is more Hawaiian.

But both forms of exercise are valuable, and you should make your own choice.

PASSIVE FUN ON THE BEACH

All of this talk of exercise and daring sportsmanship can becloud the real health secret of the water's edge: fresh air, fun and frolic.

Old-time Hawaiians fish and gather seaweed. They catch crabs, look for shells and collect coral and driftwood.

Younger adults bring guitars and sing. They picnic and party. Some go out in canoes for a paddle. Others play horseshoes or throw a Frisbee or put up a volleyball net between two palm trees.

BETTER CIRCULATION; BETTER COORDINATION; BUSTLINE IMPROVEMENT; WEIGHT CONTROL. Occasionally, a new device surfaces to provide still another beach-side game—like the Playbuoy, a mainland import already used by Y's, hotels, the Boy Scouts and professional teams. A spindle rides two strings and is sent back and forth between two players who stand about 50 feet apart. A sharp pulling apart of the handles attached to the strings sends the spindle or buoy traveling at a high velocity. Its users claim that it is great for circulation and coordination. Women say it improves their bustline and helps control weight.

Children at the beach feed the birds, chase each other and build sand castles. This latter activity is infectious; people of all ages admire their handiwork and get involved. All types of realistic carvings result, from sunning nudes to 60-foot dragons.

Now the activity has been dignified by the Annual Great Hawaiian Sandcastle Event, sponsored by no less than the Department of Architecture at the University of Hawaii.

At the end of the day, whatever the tide has not washed away is leveled for a new start tomorrow.

No one of these beach-side activities can be called a Hawaiian and Polynesian health secret. But all of them together spell out one of the most important secrets of them all: Get outdoors. Be it hillside, park, mountain or beach. Be active. Have fun.

Do this every chance you get. If you do not have the chance, create it. You are creating a chance for a longer, healthier life.

9

Polynesian Ways to Protect Yourself Against the Killing Effects of Stress

This chapter can be your vacation in Hawai'i. It is a fun chapter because fun is one of the health secrets of Hawai'i.

Stress is a killer. It is killing people every day. The antidote to stress is fun.

Get more enjoyment into your life and you will have a longer life to enjoy.

In this chapter, we examine Hawaiian fun to remind you of what you can do wherever you live to let fun dissolve stress. Here are some of the things you will discover:

GARDENING AS THERAPY   PROFESSIONAL MASSAGE
FLOWER ARRANGING   HEALTHIER MUSIC
A NERVE FOOD   MUSICAL THERAPY
SOURCES OF CALCIUM   DANCE THERAPY
SOURCES OF MAGNESIUM   FLOWER THERAPY
MAKING THINGS RIGHT   THERAPY IN CELEBRATION
RELEASE OF STRESS   STRESS-DISSOLVING ACTIVITIES
SELF-MASSAGE   THERAPY OF MIRTH

Hawai'i is a happy place.

The spirit of *aloha* includes so many joyous qualities—welcome, love, hospitality—that it cannot really be fully defined.

True, there are segments of the population where the spirit of *aloha* is being eroded or never really existed. But these are in the minority and, by and large, *aloha* is alive and well and living in Hawai'i.

Karl Marx once said, "Religion is the opiate of the people." There are some in Hawai'i who consider *aloha* to be the barbiturate of the people, making them oblivious to the "life is real, life is earnest" philosophy.

We are on the side of *aloha*. It may well turn out that *aloha* is the best health secret of them all.

Life is indeed real and it is indeed earnest. But the time-money syndrome should not be mistaken for all there is to life. When this mistake is made, stress dominates. It becomes a continuing strain. And it becomes only a matter of time for stress to take its toll. The toll of stress is death. And it comes through many doorways.

Just as a metal subjected to continued stress becomes fatigued and is no longer able to carry a load, so do the organs of the human body become fatigued from stress and begin to malfunction or cease to function at all.

Aloha is not a monopoly of Hawai'i. Just about everybody who visits Hawai'i not only benefits by *aloha* but takes a little *aloha* back home. Wherever life is lived at a relaxed pace, with cooperation prevailing over competition, there is a degree of *aloha*—and a lessened degree of stress.

This chapter will bring *aloha* to you, Hawaiian style. Whatever aspects of it you can adapt to your own life style will act as a life preserver for you in the ocean of stress that attempts to engulf us all.

THE ART OF BEING CALM: RESILIENCY

A group of Japanese archers are demonstrating in a Honolulu park. The 18 archery experts have come to Hawai'i from Japan at their own expense to compete with a Honolulu Zen archery club. They include the woman champion of Japan and also a 70-year-old man who holds the world record for accuracy with 92 hits out of 100.

Each Japanese archer is poised, slow in motion, expressionless and precise. For them it is a ritual. Before they begin, they perform an ancient Shinto ceremony. Then, as they ready their bows, each motion has a special meaning. This is *kyodo*, the Japanese martial art of archery.

Martial arts teach balance and maintaining composure. They acknowledge the life forces that surround us and harness them through passive awareness.

A number of martial arts are popular in Hawai'i. There must be a score of *judo* classes going on at any one time and plenty of *tai chi* classes.

The Asian influence in Hawai'i has been a good one when evaluated against stress. Theirs is a placid outlook. They appreciate the serenity of nature and like to keep in contact and in tune with her.

GARDENING THERAPY; FLOWER ARRANGING. The people here of Japanese descent are avid gardeners. They are masters in the art of creating *bonsai*, dwarfed trees and plants. And they are artists in flower arranging, *ikibana*, calligraphy, *sumi* brush painting, tea ceremony and many other arts and crafts.

These are calming activities. They are better than whiskey or tablets of Valium.

Writing in *Executive Health Report*, J. A. Gray, Ph.D., states that animal laboratory research shows that it is far better to develop ways of coping with stressful problems than to attempt to dissolve them with a pill. He states that any drug which reduces a person's anxiety also reduces his capacity to cope with stress. And the amount of alcohol that is enough to alter our emotions is also enough to befuddle our thoughts.

Stress works on our bodies to cause headaches, lack of energy, depression, ulcers, nervous rashes, high blood pressure, sex difficulties, premature aging and heart disease.

That's just for starters. Or should we say "enders." There are many more ways in which stress gets to us.

On the mainland, where the competitive drive is keener and more intense than in Hawai'i, stress is taking a heavier toll. The main tools to fight it, like relaxation seminars, alpha training and cassette programs, are making some headway.

These tools are available in Hawai'i also, where relaxation is a far more developed art than on the mainland; but the people who live in Hawai'i have also developed a special resiliency. They flow with time. They flow with good news and bad news. They flow with circumstances.

"Howzit, brah?"

"Gooood."

Lillian G., a divorcee, was on the verge of a nervous breakdown when she arrived in Honolulu from California to visit her daughter. Because she was getting on in years, meeting a new man she could marry was her all-encompassing goal in life. Each day she was more aware of her age, more concerned about her looks, and it made her more tense about her search. Men saw her as a bundle of nerves. They avoided her in droves.

Her daughter lived on the north shore of Oʻahu, away from the Waikiki and downtown "crush." Here, surfers and "hippy"-types lived, with nothing on their minds but fun.

Lillian began to double date with her daughter. She found that she was in demand among the 20 to 30 set. She forgot about how she looked. She had meaningful relationships. She became caught up in a totally different life. She dropped the old tensions and anxieties like hot potatoes. This was more like it.

After a month of this life, she decided to move to the other side of the island where she could more easily meet people of her own "set." She dressed up, but now she was a different woman. She became poised, calm and self-assured. The last we saw of her was when she returned to the mainland saying, "I'm not thinking of marriage. I'm having too much fun!"

WHY HAWAIIANS HAVE HEALTHY NERVES

Honolulu is a beehive of stress disciplines. Just about every mainland stress approach has had a practitioner introduce it in Hawaiʻi (if for no other reason than to obtain a tax deduction for his or her vacation!).

Some have "taken," notably Rolfing, Rebirthing, and Silva Mind Control (which the male partner of your team of authors teaches here). But the people who need these mainland disciplines are the ones who have not developed healthy nerves the Hawaiian way.

The Hawaiian way is through music, dance and fun. The Hawaiian way is living on "Hawaiian time," which runs a bit less stressfully than Greenwich time. The Hawaiian way is to confront stressful people situations and hug and kiss them away.

The drivers in Honolulu's traffic are among the most considerate in the world. Need to change lanes? They wave you in with a smile. Need to make a left turn? Oncoming traffic slows up. Need to cross a main artery? Each lane stops to accommodate you. Can you imagine that happening in a mainland city? Or would you ever see this bumper sticker: "Please no get mad if we slow—we run on Hawaiian time"?

For 20 million depressed, nervous and irritable Americans, the Hawaiian way seems totally foreign. Hundreds of thousands of them would rather pay $25 to $60 an hour for psychological or psychiatric therapy. Still others would rather drink away their cares and burn out their brains and livers. The rest prefer tranquilizers, such as Valium, Seconals and methaqualones. Sales of these drugs have increased some five-fold in the last stressful decade.

If you are drug-oriented, then forget the Hawaiian way, or do something that even the Hawaiians do not realize they are doing—produce healthier nerves.

TWO MINERALS THAT COMBAT STRESS

Calcium and magnesium are two important mineral supplements.

There is plenty of calcium and magnesium in the fresh fruits and vegetables that Hawaiians eat daily. The same may not be true for you. Calcium and magnesium are nerve foods.

A NERVE FOOD. Dolomite is a natural mineral composed of calcium and magnesium. It is extracted from limestone. However, it is inorganic. Plants can metabolize inorganic minerals easily, but we need to eat the plants that have done so. These are the organic minerals. For example, we would get more iron from a portion of spinach than we would get from a teaspoonful of iron filings.

Still, your nerves will benefit if you take dolomite because you will absorb some of it. There are other advantages to dolomite. It supplies calcium and magnesium in the right balance. It does not have the high amounts of phosphorus that most other sources of minerals have and which may not be needed by your body.

Other natural or organic supplements that contain calcium are bone meal, calcium lactate and oyster shell meal. Magnesium supplements are, to the best of our knowledge, inorganic, but are available at your pharmacy's vitamin counter or at your health food store.

SOURCES OF CALCIUM. Foods that contain calcium include milk, cheese and *poi*; green leafy vegetables like lettuce, broccoli, watercress and dandelion greens; sesame and sunflower seeds; almonds and walnuts; oats and millet.

SOURCES OF MAGNESIUM. Foods that contain magnesium include soybeans; nuts; those same green leafy vegetables, especially beet tops;

whole grains; the same seeds; and such fruits as figs, peaches and apples.

These are stress foods for everyone. But what is one person's stress may be another person's success.

TYPICAL STRESSFUL SITUATIONS THAT ERODE HEALTH

We keep talking about stress and its effects on health, but many people are not aware that they are under stress.

Vera F., a divorcee and associate teacher, always talked about her problems to us. She had problems with her two teenage children whom she eventually had to send to their father. She had problems with her supervisors. She had problems with her steady boyfriend. And many others in between.

Despite Vera's awareness of natural foods, she developed arthritis and gout. No amount of accepted dietary approaches seemed to help.

Then one day she asked us, "What is stress?"

"Stress, Vera," we replied, "are all those problems you have been sharing with us."

"Oh."

Vera then began to practice some relaxation exercises. But more important, she realized that her good health meant more to her than the petty frictions she was permitting to "bug" her. She shrugged them off and expanded her other interests.

Within a few weeks her joint pains had disappeared. We could tell, because her conversation changed from all about her problems to all about her new friends, hobbies and courses.

Stress is insidious. It does its dirty work quietly and often unobserved. Then the health problem hits and you ask, "Why me?"

Here are a few answers to that question—stressful life situations that might be causing you stress right now or may cause stress in the future:

Marital disputes	Pregnancy
Divorce	Child rearing
Separation	Accident
Family death	Unrealized goals
Family sickness	Robbery
Rivalry	Attack
Competition	Income problems

Bankruptcy	Pain
Job dissatisfaction	Jealousy
Intoxication	Overweight
Excessive smoking	Sexual conflict
Drugs	Sexual fears
Neighbors	Sexual dissatisfaction
Debts	Academic load
Mistakes	Time deadlines
Gambling	Guilt
Deprivation	

Note that all of these can be happening either to you or to someone else, and yet they can still cause stress in you.

These problems all exist as causes of stress in Hawai'i. Yet they do not "reach" the people here with the same impact as they do on the mainland. Here are some of the reasons why.

THE HAWAIIAN WAY TO MAKE THINGS RIGHT

Hawaiian words are often long and difficult to pronounce. Like *ho'o ponopono*. This word can save your life. You do not even have to pronounce it for it to go to work for you. All you have to do is to understand what it means, then apply its concept in your life.

MAKING THINGS RIGHT. Ho'o ponopono means to set right, to correct, to make right. It usually takes place within a family. But it could also refer to a team, a staff or a group of neighbors. The way things are "set right" is through prayer, discussion, confession, repentance and mutual forgiveness.

It is one of the most successful stress relievers in all of the many cultures of the world.

Before the *Hokule'a* left on its famous trip to Tahiti in 1977, there was jealousy between the *haoles* (Caucasians) and Hawaiians, friction between the captain and the crew and resentment over the financial hardships experienced by those who were making sacrifices in order to make the historic voyage successful.

Before the boat set sail to navigate by the stars on this long sea voyage, the crew got together to talk out their feelings. There were angry voices, nettled nerves and bitter expressions. But then, after an hour or so of this, a hush came over everyone. All had had their say. The air was cleared. They rose as one body and hugged each other. In twos, threes and fours, they hugged each other.

Ho'o ponopono was completed.

The voyage was a historic success.

The basic structure of *ho'o ponopono* is confession, discussion, forgiveness. Usually, it occurs within a small family or company group. If a larger group is involved, it does not work as well because one-to-one confrontations are needed in order to de-charge the stressful aspects of the interpersonal relationships.

Usually one person leads the *ho'o ponopono*. It is usually begun and followed by prayer. One's religious persuasion does not matter. Even an agnostic can meditate or commune with his or her higher self.

Next, the leader or a principal in the problem makes a statement about the problem to be solved or the condition which the participants wish to prevent from getting worse.

A frank discussion then takes place regarding conduct, emotion or attitude. This includes self-scrutiny as well as criticism, all in the spirit of total truthfulness and sincerity.

To control disruptive emotions, all remarks, replies and reactions are channeled through the leader, who may also question participants.

Next comes a confession of a wrongdoing, a grudge or a feeling of resentment, followed by a time for individual prayers or confession.

Arrangements are immediately made for restitution on the spot or at some agreed future time, if property or material possessions are involved.

Now the individuals are ready for mutual forgiveness, hugs, handshakes, embraces and a final prayer.

RELEASE OF STRESS. Ho'o ponopono is a magnificent release of stress. It is a health secret of the Hawaiians. Other Polynesian people also believe in settling problems quickly and openly, either through their chiefs or by some other method. But the Hawaiian *ho'o ponopono* is adaptable anywhere.

Western psychology emphasizes analysis, causality, assertiveness and awareness.

Eastern psychologies emphasize nonattachment, letting go, yielding and meditation.

Hawai'i, where East meets West, seems to combine the two.

We urge you to do a *ho'o ponopono* this week. When you carry any grudge or animosity or peeve within you, it tugs at some organ or system until it affects your health. This effect is an expensive price to pay for that peeve.

Talk it out with someone.

"I've had something on my mind. Can we talk about it?"

"Can I get something off my chest?"

"Something you are doing bothers me. Maybe it's my fault. Do you want to hear about it?"

This should be done in person, not over the phone or by letter. The conversation must "pull no punches." Everything has to be laid on the table. Then, with confession and discussion over with, the stage is set for adjustment in behavior and forgiveness; you hug or shake hands.

Congratulations! You have just avoided an ulcer, a heart attack or some other equally debilitating physical effect of an emotional problem.

RELEASING STORED-UP STRESS IN THE BODY

The expression "up tight" is remarkably descriptive. Therapists now realize that the body is a storehouse of stress effects. Each little incident where someone gives you "a pain in the neck" adds more rigidity to the neck muscles. Each little incident where the load of responsibility makes you feel like you are carrying the world on your back adds more twist to the tissues around the spine.

The Hawaiians knew this.

The *lomi* stick may be found only in museums now, but it was a practical way of giving yourself a massage and releasing stored-up stress. You might write to Kona Crafts, Kailua-Kona, Hawai'i 96740. When we last checked, *lomi* sticks were available for $7.00.

The *lomi lomi* massage is still administered by licensed therapists who know this technique. It includes walking on the back of the client as he or she lies on the ground. After Hawaiians use the *lomi* stick, they usually take a green drink, such as parsley juice, as a restorative.

All of this goes backward and forward in time. Ancient Chinese teachers massaged the central spine and the meridian lines on either side, known as the acupuncture *YU* points. Modern America has Rolfing, a deep tissue massage that releases old stressful "memories."

SELF-MASSAGE. We do not advise you to invite someone to walk up and down your back. But modern versions of the *lomi* stick are available and a self-massage, *lomi* style, may be just what you need.

Any massage stick that you spot in a novelty store is worth a try. We are not talking about a back scratcher, which looks like an extension of your own arm. A massage stick is usually a bent piece of wood or a roller.

One item that is available through direct mail is the MA-roller.* You lie on it on the floor and roll back and forth. It releases tensions and blockages of the normal flow of health and energy.

PROFESSIONAL MASSAGE. If you have access to a masseur or masseuse at an athletic club, health spa, hotel or in private practice, treat yourself to a massage. It will be like taking a weekend off from stress.

HEALTH BENEFITS OF MUSIC AND DANCE

The strains of Hawaiian music are so liltingly unique that they instantly strike a note of recognition wherever in the world they are heard.

HEALTHIER MUSIC. Experiments done with the brain's electroencephalogram (EEG) show that when hard rock music is played there is usually an increase in brain wave frequency. When soothing, Hawaiian-type music is played, there is a slowing down of brain wave frequency.

A slower brain wave frequency indicates a relaxed body and mind—a healthy state.

Plants grow toward symphonic music and away from fast beat, rock-type music. Plants "know" what is good for them.

Music—the *ukulele*, the guitar, the nose flute and the hula—has always been part of the Hawaiian life style, perhaps more so than in any other part of Polynesia.

It does not require a party. It does not require a *lu'au*. It does not have to be any kind of special occasion. Someone will strum. Voices will sing together. Someone will get up and do a hula or, even seated, tell the story of the music with their hands.

It could happen at a picnic, in your living room, at the beach, waiting for a bus, driving in a car.

---

*Great Earth Healing, Inc., 660 Elm Street, Montpelier, Vermont 05602.

Music is in the Hawaiian blood and it is infectious. Whoever comes to live in Hawai'i begins to know its music.

"I want to go back to my little grass shack in Kealakekua Hawai'i."

"Hawai'i Pono'i" (Hawai'i's own).

"There's an island across the sea—beautiful Kaua'i—and it's calling, just calling to me . . ."

"Puamana, Ku'u home in Lahaina . . ."

When we came to live in Hawai'i, our son Dennis was 13 years old. He listened to Hawaiian music played on the beach at Waikiki every Sunday night, led by an octogenarian man of Hawaiian blood named Papa Dave. When Dennis expressed an interest in playing the *ukulele*, we bought him one, plus a few lessons from Papa Dave. Inside of a few months, he was up there entertaining with the rest of them, and gradually acquired a pleasant singing voice and a repertoire of 50 songs in the Hawaiian language.

Dennis arrived here as a child and after ten years of Hawaiian food, outdoor life and music, he has grown to be a healthy, strapping man crowding six feet.

MUSICAL THERAPY. Music dissolves stress at its starting point. Use it yourself. Become addicted to symphony music, popular music, classical music, Oriental music or Hawaiian music. Sit down. Turn on the radio. It will be easy if you keep it tuned to a classical or popular music station, usually FM. When you get home from the usual stressful day, turn on the music.

DANCE THERAPY. Dancing is also therapeutic. Again, it does not have to be the hula. Thousands of men and women do the ancient hulas in Hawai'i. The movement of the hips is secondary to the movement of the hands in this dance, because the hula is a way of telling a story. There was neither writing nor reading in the old days. Hawaiians passed on their legends and told about their local heroes using a sign language with their hands.

Hula is the language of the heart, and hula is therefore the heartbeat of the Hawaiian people.

The female member of this writing team has performed the hula in public at many important gatherings. She teaches it and keeps studying it herself. It gives her joyous moments, dissolving the stress of writing deadlines.

She took hula lessons while she was still on the mainland. There may be a hula teacher near you. If not, any kind of dancing will do. If you do not dance now, take dancing lessons. Arthur and Kathryn Murray, founders of the Arthur Murray Dance Studios who recently celebrated their 54th anniversary, live in Hawai'i. They love to dance and are frequently seen on the dance floors of Honolulu night spots.

When the Royal Hawaiian Hotel initiated tea dancing in 1979, 500 people showed up. At the present writing, Del Courtney's band is still playing to a full house every Friday afternoon.

The Hawaiian life style is on a musical wavelength. Does that kill Hawaiians or cure them? You know the answer to that, and if you want to raise your level of health, too, put more music and dancing into *your* life.

THE ROLE THAT FLOWERS CAN PLAY IN HUMAN HEALTH

When you get off the plane in Honolulu, someone may place a flower garland over your head and around your neck. It is called a *lei*. It is the symbol of *aloha*.

Usually made of ginger flowers, plumeria or vanda orchids, the flower *lei* is given as a gesture of friendship, welcome and recognition. For each person the *lei* has a special meaning: a sweetheart, a baby, a dear friend, a song, a poem.

Dignitaries coming to Hawai'i are often bedecked with so many *leis* by their admirers that they can hardly turn their heads.

Flowers are everywhere in Hawai'i. Every season of the year you can see flowers on trees, bushes and shrubs wherever you go.

Something happens inside you when you see a flower. That is why they are on restaurant tables. That is why they are gifts of romance. That is why they fill sickrooms.

Music, dance, flowers. Put them together and they add up to something we have no word for. If there was a word meaning the opposite of "stressful" in the dictionary, that word would be the right umbrella term for music, dance and flowers.

FLOWER THERAPY. Flowers, like music and dance, are therapeutic. They help Hawaiians and other Polynesians to live longer.

A method of obtaining the essence of flowers was devised in Great

Britain and found to be helpful with different mental and emotional problems. Hawaiians use several flowers as healing herbs—we have already mentioned these—but Hawaiians never take flowers for granted. They wear them in their hair, pin them on their clothes, arrange them in their homes, give them as gifts and admire them locally whenever and wherever blossoms cross their paths.

Hawaiians are not unique in this regard, at least not in their healthy respect for the health-promoting factor in flowers. While they gave *'ilima* blossoms to pregnant women to ensure that the birth canal was lubricated, and later to ensure a plentiful supply of milk, and when they strengthened the infant's eyes by blowing the petals of the *'ilima* across its face, people of Turkey used the *Hermodactyl* flower as a cathartic. The people of Ceylon grew the orchid *Dendrobium* on every roof for its healing properties. The Hottentots of South Africa ate the flower called *Mesembryanthemum* as a remedy against exhaustion. And the people of Great Britain used agrimony for liver trouble, violets for headaches and gentian for ulcers.

We have already listed some flower remedies used by the Hawaiians and Polynesians and available to you on the mainland.

Now we would like to suggest that flowers in general deserve a greater role in your life. They deserve a place on your desk, on your dining table, in your kitchen, in your bedroom—even if it is only one blossom.

Corsages should not be reserved only for formal occasions but should be worn more often to bring relaxation and beauty to any occasion.

The flower in a man's suit jacket buttonhole should be seen more often and be the subject of small talk, fragrance and admiration.

Flowers bear the essence of life. They radiate color and light. They are a Hawaiian and Polynesian health secret that doctors cannot explain but nevertheless support in every hospital.

They may be expensive at some times of the year, but there is always some blossom that is in greater supply than others even in the dead of winter, because of a shipment from the south or from Hawai'i, or because of a local greenhouse supply.

Make your own window "hothouse." Have flowering plants inside your house and outside. Keep flowers growing—and they may help to keep you going.

OTHER WAYS THAT HAWAIIANS DEFUSE STRESS

Are you beginning to get a picture of fun-loving Hawaiians enjoying their music, singing their songs, dancing their hula and wearing flower *leis*?

As you hold this picture in your mind, remember, too, that these are the same people who buy and sell in the hectic stock and bond market, who own busy retail shops, who are in the high-pressure advertising and public relations business, who wholesale competitively, and who have the same stressful interpersonal relationships as you have on the mainland.

So the music, songs, dances and flowers are acting on the same stage as stress. Against them, stress does not have a chance. Music, song and flowers upstage stress every time. Stress cannot cohabit with fun. When fun confronts stress, fun wins hands down every time.

Hawaiians and other Polynesian people have a natural understanding of this. They enjoy their fun. *Lu'aus*, parties, banquets and festivals are continuous. The calendars of forthcoming events are replete with cultural pageants, historical observances and just plain games.

On May Day, Hawaiians hold a *lei* contest and celebrate with hula dance demonstrations in the big outdoor Shell. May 5 is Boys' Day, when a fish-shaped kite is hung outside for each boy in the family, borrowing from the Japanese custom using carp. Prince Kuhio Day in March honors Hawai'i's first delegate to Congress with ancient chants. King Kamehameha, who united the islands, is honored on his June birthdate with a parade. Flower-bedecked floats and horseback riders represent each of the islands vying good-naturedly with each other.

From the Japanese come the Cherry Blossom Festival and the *Bon* Dance. From the Chinese come New Year's Festivals with fireworks and dragon dances. From the Samoans come Flag Day celebrations.

Hawai'i welcomes in the New Year on December 31 like nowhere else. Fireworks begin all over the islands in the afternoon, reach a deafening crescendo at midnight and continue through dawn. This may be a way for some people to relieve stress but it causes stress for others, especially domestic animals and zoo animals, with a number of casualties reported each year. It is also definitely not a health-promoting activity from the point of view of the dense smoke that it produces, a danger to older people and those with respiratory problems.

THERAPY IN CELEBRATION. But its intensity is indicative of the Hawaiian zest for celebration, a quality that does indeed dissolve stress.

When you analyze it, it is the celebration of life. It derives from cultural heritage and historical excuses, but its existence does not depend on these factors.

Nor need your celebration.

You can symbolize your enjoyment of life by taking part in festivities, fun and frolic and, in the process, be giving yourself an effective dose of life-prolonging, anti-stress medicine.

Go to a carnival.

Take part in the county fair.

Have an Independence Day picnic.

Encourage your Chamber of Commerce or local historical group to sponsor a meaningful city, town or village event. Get local artists to display publicly—in Honolulu they do so every Saturday and Sunday at a long fence that separates a park from the zoo. Have the school band perform publicly in the park on Sunday afternoons.

STRESS-DISSOLVING ACTIVITIES. Participate more actively and frequently in whatever cake bakes, square and folk dancing, or other events are taking place in your community. These take you out of the tense climate of serious survival and into the relaxed, carefree climate where survival is more likely to be assured.

THE CHILDREN OF HAWAI'I

In Hawaiian schools, education takes a back seat to life. Time gets insulted. Attendance records are a farce. The English language is fractured. Many high school graduates can barely read and write.

Yet they survive. They grow up healthy. They make money. They get married. They raise fun-loving children. Some even grow rich and famous.

And they all live longer.

Here is the way an eighth grader, Mimi W., described his philosophy of life. The title of this short poem is "Bum By," which translates from the pidgin as "bye and bye":

My mada say, "Clean your room befor I bash in your face!"
I say, "Bum By."
My fada say, "Do wat your mada say!"
I say, "Bum By."
I stay 14 years old and still in da numba two grade.
My mada say, "Eh, son, when you goin grow up?"
I say, "Bum By."

Hawaiian children swing on tree limbs from elementary grades to high school grades. They horse around. They laugh and play games their mainland peers have long since left behind at that age.

When African tulip trees blossom, they pick clusters of the still-green flowers filled with nectar, bite off the tips of the firm green pods—and have instant squirt guns.

Hawaiian children laugh a lot.

THERAPY OF MIRTH. It is now known that when we laugh our nervous system takes a holiday. The medical valve of mirth may have been known about for hundreds of years, but now mirth is being taken seriously. It is very real therapy.

A recent survey of nervous breakdowns in Europe showed that Ireland had fewer incidences than any European country. The reason offered was that Ireland was the least industrialized, but the Irish had a good laugh at that. They knew it was because of their wit and persiflage. There is more laughter in Ireland than anywhere in Europe.

When we laugh, we take a momentary holiday from stress. The diaphragm, moving up and down vigorously, empties and fills our lungs, expelling stale air and sending oxygen surging to tiny capillaries that have been getting short-changed. Laughing promotes a feeling of well-being, largely because it is stress-free while it frees us of stress.

Hawaiians are childlike at any age. This is their heritage and their wisdom. They are children of the rainbow.

10

Basic Health Recipes
of the Hawaiians
and Polynesians

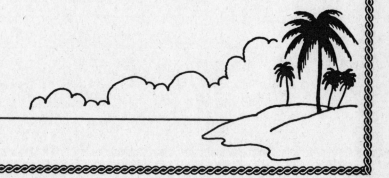

Knowing what foods are the healthiest to eat is only part of the story. You need to know how to prepare these foods for maximum enjoyment and benefit.

In this chapter, we take a trip through Polynesia to see firsthand the "what" and the "how."

And in the process we discover:

LONGEVITY FOOD

CHILDREN'S HEALTH DRINK

HEALTH BREAKFAST

LOW-STARCH GRAVY THICKENER

NUTRITIOUS DESSERT

A SPECIAL BREAD

THE NUT NAMED NIU

LOW-SUGAR DESSERT

MARSHMALLOW SUBSTITUTE

TREE "VEGETABLE"

SOUP TONIC

FISH HAWAIIAN-STYLE

CHOLESTEROL-FREE PROTEIN

FRESH = ALIVE

QUANTITY FOODS

SAMOAN HEALTH RECIPES

SAMOAN HEALTH DRINK

TAHITIAN BEAUTY FOOD

TAHITIAN HEALTH DESSERT

MAORI HEALTH BREAD

NEW ZEALAND FRUIT FAVORITE

NEW ZEALAND GRAIN FAVORITE

ORGANIC FARMING BENEFITS

FIJIAN HEALTH FAVORITES

TONGAN FAVORITE

The early Polynesians crossed vast areas of the Pacific Ocean without succumbing to scurvy or the other health problems that plagued later European explorers.

The foods that made possible their incredible voyages across the world's largest ocean, and from which they derived their sturdy health and vigor, are the very foods that we have described in previous chapters—staples of the South Pacific.

These staple foods—such as the sweet potato, banana, yam and coconut—and the plants from which they grow were carefully wrapped in leaves and reeds and stored in the holds of the ancient double-canoes to nourish these intrepid navigators who made their way against overwhelming odds, their combined strength pitted against the mighty ocean, to the scattered tropical islands of the South Pacific.

In this chapter, we share recipes old and new for preparing these vital foods in tasty ways using ingredients you already have in your kitchen.

SAVORING A "TREASURE" OF KING TUT

There is evidence that Egyptian ships were among those first explorers of the South Pacific. One of the oldest of cultivated vegetables was feasted upon in ancient Egypt and, because it is found in many islands of the South Pacific, there is a possibility that it could have been brought by the Egyptians.

This "treasure" of the land of King Tut is *taro*.

Botanists call it *Colocasia esculenta*. Hawaiians call it *kalo*. If you have visited Hawai'i, you have tasted it as *poi*.

A smaller, fresh *taro* root is available in Oriental food markets located in Chinese or Japanese neighborhoods of larger cities. But most supermarkets stock the mashed roots—*poi*—in jars and some stock it in its dehydrated or powder form.

The Hawaiians depended largely on *poi* before new foods were introduced, first by visiting Polynesians and then by the succession of visitors who followed Captain Cook. Some ate as much as 10 pounds of *poi* a day and grew into huge specimens of towering strength.

In the old days, the chefs of Polynesia would first cook the *taro* root. Then, after peeling it, they would mash it with a heavy stone pestle.

Water was added until it reached its proper consistency. When it could be eaten with one finger—because it was so stiff—it was called "one finger *poi*," but as it loosened with additional water, more fingers would be needed and so there was also "two finger *poi*" and "three finger *poi*." Finally, it was placed in a calabash, hung from the rafters and permitted to ferment for a day or two.

Fermentation is the secret.

LONGEVITY FOOD. We have already pointed out the nutritional advantages of *poi*, how it is loaded with calcium and B vitamins, how it is a perfect first food for babies, strengthening teeth and bone structure, how it is nourishing for the elderly and others who require soft diets. However, the health and longevity secret of this food is hidden in its fermented state.

Many wonder foods of the world that have been credited with a longevity factor, such as cheese and wine in France and yogurt in central Europe, have been fermented foods. Acidophilus milk is fermented.

We do not know why the fermentation process provides a nutritional boost, but why argue with success?

Here is how to ferment *poi* which you have bought in a jar or which you have purchased dehydrated and have reconstituted with water:

> *Place* poi *in a bowl and cover with one-half inch of water. Top with a protective wrap or paper towel. Let stand at room temperature. Taste in one day. If you prefer it more sour, let stand another day. Once the taste is right, stabilize by storing in refrigerator.*

Poi is not the best tasting of foods, so here are some ways to combine it with other foods.

POI POINTERS AND RECIPES

Hawaiians eat *poi* with fish. It can be delicious once you've acquired the taste, since it has more flavor than plain mashed potatoes. Here are some more interesting ways you can make use of it.

CHILDREN'S HEALTH DRINK. Your kids (*keikis* in Hawaiian) will love a "Keiki Kocktail." Blend ¾ cup of *poi* (reconstituted according to the directions on the jar) with 4½ cups of milk. Sweeten with honey (to your *keiki's* taste), flavor with vanilla. Add a dash of nutmeg. Pour into glasses partly filled with cracked ice. "Yummy, mummy," six *keikis* will say.

HEALTH BREAKFAST. Or try it for a nutritious breakfast. Put 1 cup of *poi* in a cereal bowl. Mix in 1 tablespoon of honey and stir in milk or cream to desired thickness.

LOW-STARCH GRAVY THICKENER. Poi is a great thickener for gravy in your stews, even in *Boeuf Bourguignon*. It has no floury taste. In fact, it's undetectable and it will add extra nutrition to any dish you prepare.

NUTRITIOUS DESSERT. For sweet-toothers, here's one of our favorite desserts:

Coconut Custard Poi

Sugar cane was the Hawaiians' only sweet and they rarely used eggs, so you know this is a modern dish.

½ C undiluted *poi*
3 eggs
⅓ C honey
1 small can unsweetened coconut milk (1½ C)

Blend all ingredients by hand or in electric blender. Pour into oven-proof dish set in shallow pan of hot water. Cook at 360 degrees for a half-hour. Chill and serve.

A SPECIAL BREAD. Here's another way to use *poi*.

Polynesian Poi Bread

8 ozs. reconstituted *poi*
1 C whole wheat flour
7 T honey
1 t cinnamon
1 t baking soda
2 slightly beaten eggs
½ C salad oil
1 t almond, rum or vanilla flavoring
½ C chopped walnuts or dried coconut
½ C raisins

Mix flour, honey, baking soda and cinnamon together.
Add combined eggs, flavoring and oil to mixture. Stir in
poi and add the rest of the ingredients. Bake in greased
pan for 45 minutes at 350 degrees. Makes one loaf.

MILKING HEALTH FROM THE COCONUT

The far-ranging Polynesians always brought coconuts on their voyages, both for the duration of the trip and to plant on arrival at their destination. Frequently the trees were already there, coconuts having floated to shore and rooted. This was like having Mother Nature greet them with a "home-cooked" meal.

THE NUT NAMED NIU. The Polynesians used every part of the coconut. The nut, of course, made food and drink. The shell was used for bowls and rudimentary spoons. The oil was used to protect the skin. And even the leaves, or fronds, of the tree were woven into baskets or hats, and plaited into loops and balls for a game called *pala'ie*.

You climb into a car, not up a tree, to get your coconuts. And when you return from the supermarket with them, you use a hammer and nail to make holes in the "eyes" and pour off the liquid. We have explained how the easiest way to open a coconut is to place it in an oven pre-heated to 375 degrees for 20 minutes, then wrap it in a towel and crack with a hammer.

There is a thin brown skin between you and the white meat. This is edible, but if you prefer, you can remove it with a vegetable peeler.

You can eat the white coconut meat on the spot. It is delicious and nutritious. But to add versatility to this food, you need to convert the meat into a puree or milk. Here is how:

Coconut Milk

Cut meat into small chunks. Add enough boiling water to
cover. Grate in electric grater, meat chopper or blender.
Drain liquid through cheesecloth. Use at once or freeze.

Hawaiians add this coconut milk to cooked chicken, fish and taro leaves. Other Polynesians mix it with breadfruit, sweet potatoes and bananas.

You can save some of the white meat for grating in your blender. Then use the grated coconut as a topping for desserts.

LOW-SUGAR DESSERT. In addition to the coconut custard *poi* described above, coconut can be used to make a pudding. An ancient favorite, this pudding is still popular today and a tradition at *lu'uas*. Its tropical sweetness needs a minimum of sugar or other sweetener.

Haupia

1   C coconut milk
1   t cornstarch (the Hawaiians use arrowroot powder)
2   T sugar (maximum, try less)
1½ T honey

Mix the cornstarch, honey and sugar, and add sufficient coconut milk to make a smooth paste. Heat the remaining milk to boiling and slowly stir in the cornstarch paste. Boil until mixture thickens, stirring frequently. Pour into a square cake pan, making a layer 2 inches thick. Allow pudding to cool. Cut it into 2-inch cubes and serve on squares of ti *leaves in Hawaiian style. Makes three servings. A softer pudding can be made by using less cornstarch.*

MARSHMALLOW SUBSTITUTE. Next time you make baked sweet potatoes with marshmallows, try topping them with coconut milk instead. Again, this recipe requires less sugar:

Coconut Creamed Sweet Potatoes

(This recipe is equally delicious using pumpkin instead of sweet potatoes.)

Grate 2 cups raw, peeled sweet potatoes. Place in uncovered oven-proof dish. Season with salt and pepper, if desired. Pour coconut milk over them and bake in moderate oven for about an hour. Top will come out crunchy. Inside it tastes like you used marshmallows.

TWO WAYS TO USE THE FRUIT OF PARADISE

Banana shoots were among the precious foodstuffs brought north in the Pacific some 500 years ago by the Hawaiian voyagers. It is not understood how several of these Hawaiian types of bananas abound also in Central and South America. This mystery takes its place alongside others that cloud the origins of the Polynesians, including the fact that the sweet potato, also carried from island to island by the Polynesians, bears a form of the Peruvian name, *kumara*, throughout Polynesia.

TREE "VEGETABLE." Just as the coconut is used both in main courses, such as chicken, and in desserts, so is the banana, the fruit of Paradise, used as a vegetable and as a dessert. Here is a recipe for each, permitting you to vary the use of this nutritious food in your daily menus.

Baked Bananas
(Maia Ho'omo'a)

Take 6 large ripe cooking bananas, wash skins and place in baking pan with just enough water to cover the bottom of the pan. Bake at 350 degrees until the skins begin to burst open. Serve hot in the skins and season with butter, salt and pepper.

Here's what to do when you have bananas ripen at the same time:

For each serving, use 1 banana, 3 T dried milk and a dash of rum or rum flavoring. Blend together and pour into wine or sherbet glasses. Chill in freezer for at least 1 hour and no longer than 2 hours. Top with a dollop of whipped cream and a touch of jam for color.

POLYNESIAN PROTEIN

Wild protein is richer in minerals than cultivated protein. The Polynesians sensed this and, although they domesticated some animals as livestock—chickens and pigs, for example—they were not naturally ranchers and herders.

On the Hawaiian islands, they found the native goose, wild duck, along with the heron, stilt and plover. This wild game and the fish of the sea provided mineral-rich protein.

SOUP TONIC. One of the fowl brought to the islands was the *moa*, a jungle chicken, found today in Malaysia. From this the Hawaiians made a chicken soup that they enjoyed for its strengthening qualities. This lends credence to the favorite cure-all remedy attributed to the Jewish mother. We are not going to give you a recipe for chicken soup, just a reminder that it could be a strengthening tonic for you.

Wild pigs and boars still abound in Hawai'i and pork remains an important source of protein on the islands. But early Europeans introduced cattle and today the second largest cattle ranch in the United States is located on the Big Island, along with many smaller ranches. A Hawaiian cowboy is called *paniolo*, and here is the cowboy's favorite beef dish, combining the best of the old and the new:

Paniolo Stew

2½ lbs. chuck roast, cubed
1½ T salad oil
1 small slice ginger
1 medium onion, diced
1 large tomato, diced
1 T salt
  dash of pepper
6½ C water
1 C *poi*
3 stalks green onion, cut in 1-inch pieces
½ small red pepper, minced

In a large pan, heat the oil; stir-fry ginger, then brown the meat. Add onion, tomato, salt, pepper and water to cover the meat. Bring to a boil; reduce heat and simmer until meat is tender. Gradually add poi, stirring to dissolve and to thicken stew. Add green onion just before serving. Serve with red pepper. 6 servings.

FISH HAWAIIAN-STYLE. In a moment, we are going to take you on a mini-visit to several islands of the South Pacific to see how Polynesians there prepare their food. But first, here are two ways in which Hawaiians prepare fish, one using salmon, the other using whatever was caught that day.

Lomi Salmon
(Kamano Lomi)

¾ lb. salted or smoked salmon
½ C onion
½ C ice water
2⅔ C sliced tomato
5 green onions with tops
1 t coarse sea salt

Clean and soak salmon 3 or more hours in cold water. Drain. Remove skin and bones and shred fish into small pieces. Smoked salmon need only be shredded. Peel and slice tomatoes. Chop onions fine. Combine tomatoes and salmon and mash with a fork. Stir in the ice water and onions. Chill thoroughly and serve in small individual bowls.

The Hawaiians prefer using only green onions. They lomi (crush) the green onions with salt using fingers or a wooden potato masher. When onions are mashed, add ¼ cup of water; then add salmon and tomatoes. 6 servings.

Fish Baked in Ti Leaves
(I'a Lawalu)

1½ lbs. fish slices *or*
2½ whole butterfish, halibut or mullet
1½ T course seasalt
Ti leaves or corn husks

Scale and clean the fish. Rub with salt. Wrap in several leaves, tying the ends together. If individual slices are used, wrap with two leaves in opposite directions. Cover

*bottom of pan with water. Place in moderate oven and
bake about one hour for whole fish or a half-hour
for individual servings.*

*Additional flavor may be added by placing a piece of
bacon, one bay leaf, slices of onion and green pepper on
each slice of fish before tying it. Serve hot in the leaves or
husks. 6 servings.*

Remember, too, that the Hawaiians loved turtle, crab, lobster and octopus. These are still being caught today but in decreasing quantities. In fact, we know of only one restaurant here that serves turtle steak. It is now illegal to catch sea turtles and this restaurant must import the turtle meat. You are probably in a better position on the mainland to buy shellfish and other fresh protein from the sea, with a large mainland fishing industry flying its products to all major markets.

CHOLESTEROL-FREE PROTEIN. Fish and shellfish are nature's purest proteins—relatively free of the cholesterol risks inherent in meat and poultry. Proteins of the sea are one of the chief Hawaiian and Polynesian health secrets, leading to good circulatory systems and longer life.

FRESH=ALIVE. The fish and shellfish are eaten as fresh from the sea as possible. We were invited for lunch to a home on the north shore of Oʻahu. After drinking some fruit juice, freshly squeezed from the fruit that was freshly picked, our host said, "Excuse me for a few minutes."

He got a spear and waded into the ocean. Soon we lost him in the breakers. In about ten minutes, he returned with four lobsters. In a few minutes they were steamed and we were enjoying the freshest seafood we had ever tasted.

The fresher the meat or fish, the better it is for you. This applies to all food. When you shop, favor fresh produce—and the closer the source to where you live, the better. Fresh food is living food, with more to contribute to your life.

THE HEALTHY FEASTS OF SAMOA

Our visits to islands of the Pacific always yield new health secrets. Some time ago, we were guests of a member of the Samoan legislature, who lived on the beach in a large home that used to be the Rain-maker Hotel, where Somerset Maugham stayed to write his famed *Rain*.

And rain it did. A festival was in progress. Rain is considered a blessing to the Polynesians, so nobody minded the torrents. It is warm rain and the air is warm, too. *Ava* was prepared and passed around during three days of open-air events.

There were singing and dancing contests, speeches by Washington big-wigs, tugs of war, parades of flower-bedecked floats, flag-raisings, feasts, prayers, cricket matches, variety shows, cocktail parties, more feasts, canoe races, another feast, the opening session of the legislature, more feasts, parties, a grand ball, movies and still more feasts.

On these feasts, the Samoans grow so husky and strong that they have the reputation wherever they go in the world of being people you ought not to tangle with.

Why is it, we asked, when Americans eat in abundance, they get fat, but when Samoans eat in abundance, they get husky and strong?

QUANTITY FOODS. The answer, of course, lies in what is eaten and how it is prepared. The fat-rich gravies and sugar-laden desserts are not on the Samoan fare. (Neither are the breads, cakes, pasta and pastries so common to the American "feast.") They eat all they want of proteins, fresh fruits and fresh vegetables.

For us the *fiafia*, the feasts, were the highlights. We were bussed to remote parts of the lovely island of Tutuila and entertained lavishly by the *Matai*, the local chiefs. We were warmly greeted with the cry of *"Talofa!"* and seated on finely woven mats on the crushed gravel floor of the open-to-the-breeze *fale*, a circular thatched building with roll-down woven blinds.

Cautioned to tuck our feet under us so they would not inadvertently point at a person of high rank, we were served, after the "high-and-talking chiefs," piles of steaming leaf-wrapped fish and meat laced with coconut milk, sliced baked *taro*, luscious tropical fruits, puddings and *poi* and drinking coconuts.

The chiefs tried to outdo one another in gracious hospitality. We were encouraged to take home all that we could not eat on the spot. At one *fiafia*, we were given woven coconut baskets called *aiiga* to carry the copious leftovers: whole chickens, hands of bananas, coconuts and breadfruit. What a "doggie bag," and what nourishing food!

Traditionally, Samoan men, like the Hawaiians of old, are the cooks. Not so our friend Imo, son of a talking-chief, who took us home to his small village of Aur. Abandoning "city clothes," he reappeared wrapped in a brilliant orange and white *lava-lava*, a crimson hibiscus tucked behind one ear, to take us on a sunset walk along the beach. Feathery clouds etched against a glowing sky as voices called out of the semi-darkness, inviting us to come and eat. Imo answered in Samoan that his wife was at home cooking our evening meal and thanked them. He explained to us that had we accepted any of the invitations, it would have been an all-night affair with a pig being slain and baked in an *umu* (an above-ground oven made of rocks in a specially-built thatched hut).

The Samoans eat at the drop of a hat and their health attests to the fact that it is not how much you eat but what you eat that counts. Of course, they are fun-loving, active people, not worrying and sedentary like most mainlanders.

After their feast, there is a fire-dance or a slap-dance by the men. There is partying, rough-housing and merrymaking. Nobody tells them to "turn the volume down."

SAMOAN HEALTH RECIPES. As it turned out, we had a quiet evening featuring delicious food prepared by our hostess. Here are three of their family recipes adapted for your use (for example, you may substitute spinach for *taro* tops):

Baked Spinach and Coconut Cream
(Palu Sami)

2½ lbs. spinach
3   C shredded packaged coconut
2   C half-and-half cream

Wash spinach and remove the tough stems. Combine the coconut and cream and allow to stand 30 minutes; simmer for 10 minutes; cool and strain through several thicknesses of cheesecloth. Squeeze out as much coconut liquid as possible, season and pour over the spinach. Salt to taste. Bake in a slow oven (300 degrees) until the spinach is tender. 6 servings.

Fish Baked in Coconut Cream
(Fa'a Laui'a)

1½ to 2 lbs. mild-flavored fish
salt
1¼ C shredded packaged coconut
¾ C half-and-half cream

Prepare coconut cream as above. Wash, scale, clean fish, keeping on head or tail. Rub salt inside and out. Place in baking dish, add the coconut cream and bake at 350 degrees for approximately one hour. 6 servings.

If you were a Samoan, you would braid a coconut frond at one end, place a *ti* or banana leaf over it, and then braid the remainder of the frond. We say, "bake at 350 degrees for an hour," and all it takes is a flick of the wrist. In Samoa, it would take hours to prepare the *umu*—an above-ground oven used to steam and roast. They boil by dropping hot white stones into gourds filled with water.

SAMOAN HEALTH DRINK. Here is a third Samoan recipe made with coconut. It is their equivalent of our "Tiger's Milk."

Banana Poi
(Poi Fa'i)

3½ C mashed, very ripe bananas
1½ T lime juice
1½ C coconut cream

Add juice to the banana pulp. Gradually, add the coconut cream, stirring. Chill and serve in sea or coconut shells. Serves 9.

A BLEND OF FRANCE AND THE TROPICS

Two thousand miles south of Hawai'i stretches French Polynesia. Here is where that symbol of the South Pacific, Tahiti, isle of dreams, lies washed by sparkling tropic seas. Here, too, some legends say the Polynesians began. And here is where reside some of the most beautiful specimens of the human race—male and female—in the world.

More than 200 years ago, the first Europeans arrived. Since then there has been a blending of races, customs and cultures. What remains of the old health and beauty ways on this popular, populous, mountainous isle shaped like a swimming tortoise? Not too long ago, we went to find out.

Greeted at the airport in Faaa—just three miles out of Papeete—by our lovely Tahitian friend, the young daughter of a prominent politician, we were whisked to their nearby hilltop home in a lush tropical setting. Though we had planned to stay in a hotel, Tiare insisted that we spend one night Tahitian-style. From our room, Tiare's own, we had a view of the azure Pacific, framed by coco-palms and banana leaves.

It was a thrill to sleep under a light, hand-made quilt patterned with breadfruit designs. The home was a blend of the tropics and the best of France. Tiare served us breakfast in the garden. She deftly sliced off the top of a husked coconut and—*voila!*—there was the champagne of the islands, that unique beverage, cool, refreshing, delicious.

Later on in our five-day stay, we sampled much of the joyous entertainment and the delectable native foods—hearts of palm right from the tree with freshly picked watercress, shellfish cooked in lime juice, rock-oysters on the half shell.

TAHITIAN BEAUTY FOOD. At dawn each day, the action begins at the "Marche Papeete," the famous market. Here's where you get the real "taste" of Tahiti, from snacks of fermented sea-snails and sugared apples marinated in wine, to the traditional handicrafts displays. Wrapped in colorful *pareau*, island beauties saunter by. Their flower-wreathed hats tilt over laughing eyes. Dark hair tumbles to slender waists. One clasps a line on which are strung, still wiggling, purple and turquoise fish. Fish is an important health and beauty source in Tahiti.

Tahitian Marinated Fish
(Ota)

Raw fish is "cooked" in lime juice in this popular Tahitian dish. It is similar to Latin America's *ceviche* without the chili peppers:

1½ lbs. firm white fish
¾   C freshly squeezed lime juice
1   small onion, sliced fine
¾   C coconut milk (or substitute ¼ C olive oil and 1
      T vinegar)

The simplest way to cut raw fish is to freeze it until it is very firm. Cut into bite-sized pieces. Put into a bowl and cover with lime juice and onions. Refrigerate for several hours. Drain and add coconut milk. Stir until coated. Garnish with chopped green onions. Tahitians often serve it with finely sliced vegetables, such as carrots, green peppers, celery, etc. Serves 4.

Fruits and flowers are everywhere in Tahiti. The beauty of both nature and the people reflect from one to the other, reinforcing and regenerating.

Pass a tree, pick a fruit and bite into it. You do not have to rinse off any poison spray. Pass a shrub, pick a flower and put it behind your ear or in your hair, whether you are male or female—on the left side if you're "lookin'," on the right side if you're "tooken." And center if you're "tooken but still lookin' "!

Baked Fruits Tropical
(Poe)

TAHITIAN HEALTH DESSERT. Tahitians collect fruits and coconuts for this healthful dessert called *poe,* not to be confused with *poi.*

1 small pineapple
1 ripe mango
1 medium papaya
¾ lb. bananas
¼ C arrowroot powder
⅓ C honey
½ C coconut milk
½ t vanilla

Grease a shallow baking dish. Peel and chop fruits. Puree in blender or meat grinder. Let stand in colander

*to drain. Mix 1 cup of the juice with arrowroot powder
and stir into the fruit mixed with remaining juice. Stir in
honey and vanilla and spread evenly on baking dish.
Bake at 375 degrees for an hour. Serve chilled with
coconut milk as a sauce. Serves six.*

You can substitute fruits in season if you cannot find a mango or a papaya.

Also, you might try mixing ripe, mashed bananas with an equal amount of *poi* for another popular Tahitian dessert that packs a nutritional wallop.

MINING FOR MAORI HEALTH SECRETS

At the southernmost tip of Polynesia are the spectacular islands of New Zealand, where volcanos heat geysers and mineral springs and where the soil is rich with nutrients. Here colonists came from Great Britain to live harmoniously with the native people, who are called the Maori.

The original diet of the energetic Maori people is still popular today: fish, fowl, sweet potato, fern roots, seaweed and shellfish. But now it is augmented by foods that the British introduced: mutton, beef and marvelous cheeses.

MAORI HEALTH BREAD. We discovered that, like the American Indian, the Maoris use the edible pollen of bulrushes, or cattails, to make bread. These bulrushes grow quite profusely around marshes and along the seacoasts of the United States.

The Maoris shake the yellow pollen from the bulrushes. Each pound is mixed with a half cup of water. The mixture is then placed in an oven-proof greased dish and steamed for two hours.

Maori Corn Pudding

Here is how the Maoris make corn pudding. Perhaps the American Indians also used this recipe.

*Grate dried corn into meal. Bind with water and make
into a dough to which a little honey and a dash of cinna-*

mon have been added. Wrap in corn leaves and place in
a steamer for 2 hours.

NEW ZEALAND FRUIT FAVORITE; NEW ZEALAND GRAIN FAVOR-
ITE. Here are some modern Maori recipes, reflecting strong British influence and using contemporary ingredients and techniques. The first is a
favorite native fruit dish, the second is a popular grain recipe, and then we
have a fish chowder and Scotch-influenced scones.

Kiwi Fruit Cake

    1 bar of butter (at room temperature)
    ½ C sugar
    2 eggs
    1 C flour
    1 t baking powder
    4 ripe *kiwi* fruits

Cream butter in mixer. Beat in sugar, eggs and sifted
flour a little at a time. Add baking powder. Pour into two
greased and floured cake pans. Bake for a half-hour at
350 degrees.
Mash 3 fresh kiwis and spread between cooled layers.
Top with your favorite icing or whipped topping. Deco-
rate with slices of kiwi cut with a stainless steel or silver
knife to prevent discoloration.

Pikelet Pancakes

    1   C whole wheat flour
    1½ t double-acting baking powder
        dash of salt
    ½   C milk
    1   egg
    1   T honey
    1   bar melted butter

Sift the flour, baking powder and salt into bowl. Make a
hole in the middle and pour in the milk, egg and honey.

Gradually mix the dry ingredients into the center and stir until the batter is smooth. Do not overmix.
Heat a heavy skillet over moderate heat. Test with a few drops of water which should bubble for a couple of seconds and evaporate. Spread melted butter lightly over the skillet. Pour the batter onto the hot pan about half a tablespoon at a time. Allow each pancake to spread into a 2-inch round.
Bake until small bubbles begin to break the surface. Turn the pancakes over with a spatula and cook them for about a minute. Stack on a heated platter. Regrease the skillet and continue with the remaining batter.
Serve the pikelets hot, with the remaining melted butter, jam and whipped cream. Makes 15 to 18 2-inch pancakes.

New Zealand Fish Chowder

12 fresh oysters
1   T butter
1   T flour
    dash of cayenne pepper
    salt to taste
2   C milk
¼   C sour cream
½   T chopped chives

Chop oysters, reserving liquid. Melt butter in heavy saucepan. Stir in flour and seasonings. Add milk and oyster liquid gradually and stir. Now add oysters and simmer for about five minutes. Top with a dollop of sour cream and sprinkle with chives. Serves 3.

North Island Scones

This is one of New Zealand's most popular treats due to the large population of Scots who have settled here:

1 C milk
1 egg
1 t baking powder
½ C whole wheat flour

Sift together baking powder and flour. Beat together the egg and milk and add to flour. Drop tablespoons of batter onto greased griddle. Brown lightly on both sides. Serve hot with jam.

ORGANIC FARMING BENEFITS. We are convinced that the Maoris and their fellow New Zealanders maintain their high levels of health largely because of the richness of their soil.

Mechanized farming in the United States has depleted the soil of much of its original nutrients. What is put back is not of the same quality or in the same quantities as what is taken out.

People with garden patches can gain from the New Zealanders by learning about organic farming, using organic rather than chemical fertilizers and avoiding the use of sprays.

With a compost pit and mulching, you can add New Zealand flavor and nutrition to your home-grown vegetables and bring a serving of Polynesian health to your table.

LONG PIG NO LONGER

Once notorious for cannibalism, the Fijians are now known as dwellers of the "happy islands," fortunately for visitors (who were formerly called "long pig"). Until recently a British colony, Fiji is now an independent country composed of many islands. Their tradition says that they came from Tanganyika on the east coast of Africa. Arriving in these lush tropic isles at the edge of the Polynesian triangle, this tall, black, fun-loving race intermingled with the native Polynesians. Many Fijian customs, crafts and foods show the influence of these earlier people.

FIJIAN HEALTH FAVORITES. Like so many other places in Polynesia, a feast of welcome begins with a kava rite called *yaqona* in Fiji. This is the ceremonial drinking of the intoxicating, non-alcoholic beverage prepared from a root of the pepper family. The feast, *magiti,* is prepared in an underground oven and consists of suckling pig, plantains, sweet potato, chicken in banana leaves and various seafoods. Almost everything is flavored with *lolo*, coconut milk.

In our all-too-brief stay on Viti Levu, we were delighted with the delicious meals at our hotel, which included delectable cheeses from New Zealand, tasty local tropical fruits and yummy British-type puddings such as our favorite tapioca. Here are some recipes we collected:

Ham and Banana Roll with Cheese Sauce

4   thinly-cut slices of cooked ham
     mustard to taste
1½ T butter
4   firm bananas
1½ C grated sharp cheese

Spread slices of ham with mustard. Peel bananas and wrap in a slice of prepared ham. Brush tips of bananas with butter. Place rolls in greased shallow baking dish. Cover with cheese sauce made by adding grated cheese to your favorite white or cream sauce. Bake at 350 degrees for about 25 minutes. Serves 2.

Banana Drop Cookies

2¼ C whole wheat flour
2   T baking powder
¼   t baking soda
¾   C honey
6   ozs. room-temperature butter
2   eggs
1   C mashed bananas
1   t vanilla
½   t cinnamon mixed with
1   T brown sugar
     chocolate or carob bits (optional)

Sift together dry ingredients. Mix with next five ingre-

*dients, beating until well-blended. Sprinkle with sugar-
cinnamon mixture. Drop by tablespoons onto ungreased
cookie sheet. Bake at 400 degrees for 12 minutes. Remove at once. Makes 3-4 dozen.*

Curried Crabs Suva

Over half the population of Fiji today are Indians whom the British
brought as indentured workers into the cane fields. Hence, the curry
recipe.

1½ C crabmeat
½   C coconut milk
    salt to taste
1   clove garlic
1   small onion
½   t curry powder
    small chili or
    dash of red pepper

*Chop onion, garlic and chili fine. Pour coconut milk to
just cover bottom of pot. Bring to boil, add onion mixture and curry and cook covered for 5-7 minutes. Add
salt and crabmeat and heat, adding rest of coconut milk.
Serves 3.*

Fijian Banana Cocktail

1   banana
½   C tomato sauce or puree
½   t Worcestershire sauce
2   T lemon juice
½   t chopped green onion

*Blend one banana with tomato sauce, adding the Worces-
tershire sauce, lemon juice and green onion. Chill and
serve. In Fiji, this concoction is served in a purple-
petaled banana flower. 1 serving.*

THE LAST POLYNESIAN KINGDOM

The islands of Tonga to the South are inhabited by Polynesians who live close to the old ways. They are a kingdom with a real live king. They still make *tapa*, which they wear as wrap-around skirts fastened at the waist by soft mats and coconut fiber belts. Their economy is founded on copra and bananas and they enjoy their outdoor feasts, *kava* ceremonies, music and dancing, little touched by foreign influence. Their staple foods are similar to the other branches of the Polynesian family.

A peaceable folk today, the Tongans in the 18th and 19th centuries carried on battling feuds with their not-too-distant neighbors of Samoa, Fiji and Melanesia.

Lupulu

TONGAN FAVORITE. Tongans use *taro* tops but you can substitute fresh spinach leaves. It is a delicious dish and easy to prepare.

1 can corned beef
1 large piece heavy-duty aluminum foil
1 can coconut milk (1½ C)
1-2 T chopped green onions
1 bunch spinach

Wash spinach and shake dry. Spread leaves out to cover the foil. Place the corned beef in the center of the leaves and sprinkle with the onions. Turn up the edges of the foil and pour coconut milk over all. Wrap and seal into a package, taking care not to spill the coconut milk. Bake in a 350 degree oven for 45 minutes. Serves 3-4.

11

Island Foods and
How to Prepare Them
for Maximum Nutrition

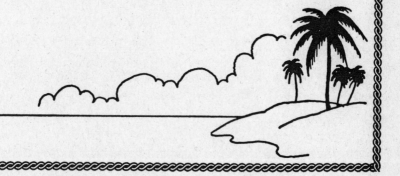

Hawai'i's people today enjoy food from many lands, prepared in many styles. One thing they all have in common is that the nutrients are never upstaged by sugar, starch and animal fats.

In this chapter, we observe the arrival of each culture and extract the best from among their classic recipes and modern adaptations, gaining in the process knowledge about:

AVAILABILITY OF
    INGREDIENTS

NUTRITION-RETAINING
    UTENSILS

VITAMIN AND MINERAL
    RETENTION

ORIENTAL PREPARATION
    TECHNIQUE

CHINESE-STYLE FISH

CHINESE PROTEIN SOUP

CHINESE SALAD

CHINESE AMBROSIA

KEY JAPANESE INGREDIENTS

LOW-FAT FRYING

SLIMMING DISH

DOUBLE PROTEIN RECIPE

ENERGIZING SALAD

WONDROUS LEAF

UNUSUAL SOUP

FOOD ADDITIVE

SEA VEGETABLE DESSERT

DESSERT WITHOUT
    SWEETENING

JAPAN'S NO. 1 HEALTH FOOD

PROTEIN SNACK

HEALTHFUL RELISH

POWER-PACKED SEED

FERMENTATION FOR
    LONGEVITY

HIGH-PROTEIN FILIPINO
    DISHES

INEXPENSIVE NUTRITION

BALANCED ENERGY BOOSTER

O'ahu, the name of the island where Honolulu and Waikiki are located, means "meeting place." Although Hawai'i has been a state now for over 20 years, its three million visitors, even though they are mostly Americans, have not been "meeting" here for long enough on their two-week vacations to materially affect the islands, their customs, the people—or their health.

O'ahu, once the meeting place for the people of the Hawaiian Island chain, is now the meeting place for the cultures of the world, chiefly the cultures of the Pacific basin.

Hawai'i is not a steak and potato place. It is not a hamburger and hot dog place. It is a crack seed, shave ice, *tofu, saimin, dim sum, malassadas* and *lumpia* place.

The food that modern Hawaiians thrive on today is affected by the people who have brought to the islands their customs, celebrations, traditions, dress, culinary arts and the wisdom to stay dynamic and healthy.

Early lava carvings on the Big Island, purportedly of Chinese origin, date back to 2000 B.C. But the first large contingent of Chinese people arrived in Hawai'i in 1852, and for 30 years they were the major labor force used by American pineapple and sugar interests.

Pooling family resources, the Chinese opened shops and businesses. Today, people of Chinese ancestry hold some of the highest positions in government and business on the islands, and their ways of cooking are prized as among the tastiest and healthiest.

We will be looking at the contributions of several cultures to the health of the islands, but because the Chinese have a knack for retaining most of the nutrition in the food they prepare, we will start with them.

HOW TO BE A CHINESE CHEF

Every large town or city in the United States has at least one Chinese restaurant, attesting to the unique taste and enjoyability of Chinese cuisine.

In addition to Chinese, Honolulu has about 20 more nationalities represented among its restaurants, but the Chinese restaurants dominate, even though the people of Chinese origin here are outnumbered by the Japanese ten to one.

AVAILABILITY OF INGREDIENTS. It is easy to cook the Chinese way. Basic ingredients are readily available in supermarkets and Oriental specialty stores. These include soy sauce *(shoyu* or *tamari)*, peanut oil, fresh ginger root, water chestnuts, bamboo shoots, bean sprouts (sprout your own) and spices. You may occasionally find Chinese vegetables in your local market, such as Chinese cabbages, and certainly snow peas are widely distributed in frozen form.

Besides the cleaver, ladle, strainers and casseroles you already have in your kitchen, you will also need a large skillet if you don't already own a *wok*. This is a large bowl-like metal pan which is the basic Chinese cooking utensil.

NUTRITION-RETAINING UTENSILS. Chinese cooking is done *fast over* high heat. We emphasize *fast*, because cooking never adds to nutrition. In fact, it can destroy certain vitamins and minerals. We emphasize *over*, because the food is held above the heat by the curve of the wok, not directly on the heat by a flat pan.

VITAMIN AND MINERAL RETENTION. Furthermore, the Chinese do not soak the food in cooking water. Water dissolves vitamins and minerals and some of the best nutrition in American food goes down the drain with the used cooking water.

Some of the time you save in cooking the Chinese way is lost in preparation. There is much slicing and pre-cutting. This should be done as close to cooking time as possible to retain freshness.

ORIENTAL PREPARATION TECHNIQUE. Stir-frying is the Chinese way. A little oil is heated in the wok or skillet. The longer-cooking pieces of food, such as meat, go into the skillet first. These are stirred over a high heat, turned over, and stirred some more.

Next, vegetables are added and stirred.

Now the heat is reduced, broth is added, and the skillet or wok is covered. In a few minutes, you can add a little arrowroot powder or cornstarch to thicken the broth. Do this by dissolving it first in soy sauce, wine or a little water.

Your Chinese way of cooking results in a delicious dish with the color and texture of its ingredients delightfully preserved and with little or no loss of vitamins and minerals.

It is said that there was once a Chinese emperor who asked his wise men to research and discover how his people could best be nourished. You now have their findings. This is the way they maintain the food juices with a proper balance of protein and vegetable carbohydrate.

NUTRITIOUS CHINESE DISHES

Now for some healthful Chinese recipes, first using the wok.

Poached Fish in Sweet-Sour Sauce

CHINESE-STYLE FISH. Every culture has its favorite sweet-sour dish. This one is popular in south China. Fish should be scaled and cleaned, but leave on the head and tail. Use sea bass, flounder, halibut or perch.

1⅔ lbs. fish
4   stalks green onion
3   slices ginger root
2   T *sake* (rice wine)
5   T sesame oil
    water to cover fish
1   t shredded red pepper
2   T chopped green pepper
6   T vinegar
4   T honey
3   T ketchup
1½ t cornstarch, dissolved in
1   T water
3   sprigs Chinese parsley

Wash fish. Mix 2 chopped stalks green onion, two slices ginger, 1 T sake. Let stand about 20 minutes. Heat large pan or wok with 1T sesame oil. Then add fish. Add wine and water to cover. When water boils again, shut off heat and let stand covered for 15-20 minutes. Remove fish and place on platter. Sprinkle with some black pepper. Heat 4 more T oil until it smokes. Then pour over fish, reserving some oil in pan. Now stir-fry 1 slice minced ginger, the rest of the green onions shredded and the red and green pepper for a couple of minutes, add the vinegar, honey, ketchup and 3 T water, and heat. Thicken with dissolved cornstarch and 1 t sesame oil. Pour sauce over fish and garnish with coriander (Chinese parsley). Serves 5.

Chinese Snow Peas

If you can't find fresh snow peas, use the frozen variety.

   2 packages frozen Chinese snow peas
   2 tender stalks celery
   2 T sesame or peanut oil
   ½ t *shoyu* (soy sauce)
   1 clove garlic

Slice celery into small pieces. Heat the oil in wok or skillet and add the clove of garlic. (Chinese chefs use a cleaver: one blow to remove skin from garlic clove, the second smashes it.) Add peas and cook, stirring for about 3 minutes. Drizzle with shoyu and serve while still crisp. Serves 4.

Peanut Butter Soup

CHINESE PROTEIN SOUP. Soups are vital to Oriental cookery. This one is an excellent source of protein and can be used for a meatless meal.

   3½ C water
   3   T peanut butter
   2   t *tahini* (sesame butter)
   ½   C water
   1½ T cornstarch
   1½ T water
   ¼   C evaporated milk

Blend the peanut butter and tahini and ½ C of the water by hand or in electric blender. Heat in the 3 C of water and bring to a boil. Dissolve cornstarch in the remaining water and thicken. Turn off heat and add evaporated milk. Stir and serve at once. 3 servings.

Chinese Cabbage Salad

CHINESE SALAD. This is a salad with a tangy flavor.

    1 Chinese cabbage
    1 T honey
    ¼ C cider or rice vinegar
    ½ C sesame or salad oil
    ½ C chopped green onions
    1 t minced fresh ginger or
    ⅛ t dried ginger
       dried red pepper to taste

Wash cabbage and cut out core. Shred and arrange on platter. Heat oil and cook onion and ginger briefly. Add pepper and blended honey and vinegar. Pour over cabbage and toss. Serves 4-5.

Lychee Almond Float

CHINESE AMBROSIA. The Chinese eat very little sweets. Here is a delicious dessert that you may have tasted and wondered how to prepare. It's great with fresh fruits in season.

    2 packages unflavored gelatin
    1 C plus 2 T water
    1 can lychee, mandarin oranges or
    ½ C diced peaches
    1 C milk
    2 T honey
    1 T almond extract

Sprinkle gelatin in the 2 T water to soften. Boil the rest of the water, add gelatin and stir until dissolved. Remove from heat. Stir in honey, milk and almond extract. Pour into flat pan and chill until firm. Dice jelly and serve with fruits and juice.

THE HEALTH ADVANTAGES OF
JAPANESE-STYLE COOKING

As pineapple and sugar plantations grew in the last century, there was a demand for more workers. The first Japanese to arrive in 1868 were soon joined by their "picture brides"—young women who agreed to come to Hawai'i to marry them through an exchange of pictures.

Today, nearly half of Hawai'i's population is of Japanese descent. *Sumo* wrestling, the tea ceremony and *Bon*-dancing—all unique to the Japanese culture—are commonplace here. *Furo* baths, flower arranging, Shinto temples and Japanese restaurants add to the panorama of island living.

The Japanese word *"gohan"* means both "rice" and "meal." So you know that rice is an important feature of the Japanese menu.

Although their method of food preparation, like the Chinese, involves cutting ingredients into small bite-sized pieces, the utensils used are not special and you can use what is already in your kitchen.

KEY JAPANESE INGREDIENTS. Japanese cooking is healthful because of the ingredients they favor, already described earlier in this book. In the menus that follow, you will find seaweed, fish and other products of the sea where minerals abound. You will find soybean products, such as *tofu, shoyu* and *miso*.

Although there is frying in fat, it is always done lightly in a way that coats but does not penetrate. You will not find french fried potatoes or doughnuts, foods that absorb and become saturated with the fat. Sesame or peanut oil are used—far healthier than the animal fats we use.

TEMPURA, SUKIYAKI AND OTHER JAPANESE DISHES

LOW-FAT FRYING. Tempura, a typically Japanese method of frying, was adapted from the method used by early Portuguese visitors to Japan. Here is one such recipe.

Shrimp Long Rice Tempura

This recipe has a simplified batter. Remember, it must be served as soon as it is cooked to retain its characteristic crispness.

> 2 lbs. fresh shrimp
> 1 bundle long rice (bean-threads)
> 2 eggs
> ¼ C cornstarch
> *shoyu* to taste
> sesame or peanut oil

Clean shrimps, slit down back leaving tails attached. Spread each one open and crisscross lightly with sharp knife. Heat the oil. Cut long rice into half-inch pieces. Beat eggs in bowl. Have cornstarch ready. Now dip shrimps first in cornstarch, then into egg mixture. Sprinkle some long rice on skin side of shrimp and slide shrimps one at a time into hot oil. Fry only on one side. Drain on folded paper towels. Serve with shoyu or tamari sauce.

The Japanese slur many of their words, and sukiyaki becomes "skiyaki." But here in Hawai'i, we call it *hekka*. It is a beef, pork or chicken dish cooked in *shoyu* with a variety of vegetables and soybean curd *(tofu)*. The hot mixture can be served in a bowl containing a raw egg. Stirred with your chopsticks, the egg quickly cooks and adds even more protein to the meal.

Chicken Sukiyaki

SLIMMING DISH. Here is a sukiyaki recipe—free of fattening fat and starchy carbohydrates.

> 2¾ lbs. chicken
> 4   C thinly sliced, canned bamboo shoots

½ C *sake* or dry white wine
2 T sesame oil
½ bunch watercress or
1 C canned water chestnuts
1 T sugar
2½ C thinly sliced, canned or soaked dried mushrooms
1½ C water (use liquid from mushrooms)
1½ C *shoyu*
1 bunch green onions with tops

Clean chicken and cut into 1-inch cubes, keeping bones. Wash and cut green onions and watercress into 2-inch lengths. Wash and soak dried mushrooms. Heat oil in heavy skillet, add one-third of the chicken and fry 15 minutes. (The Japanese custom is to prepare sukiyaki in a pan over a charcoal brazier on the table. One third is cooked at a time and then placed in individual bowls, as the second third is cooked, and so forth, so the food is hot and fresh.) Add some liquid if necessary. Now put in the sugar and shoyu. Cook 3 minutes and add one-third of the mushrooms and bamboo shoots. After 5 minutes, add one-third of the onions, watercress and sake or wine. Serve over brown rice. 8 servings.

Shabu is cooking in hot broth at the table. Our first experience with this method was at the Tokyo Hilton in Japan. Now we order it frequently at Japanese restaurants in Honolulu. It is not unlike the French *bouillabaisse*, which we had at a seaside restaurant in Cannes and which is popular in New Orleans.

DOUBLE PROTEIN RECIPE. You partake of the broth in both the French and Japanese versions, getting the benefit of the dissolved minerals and vitamins instead of pouring them down the kitchen sink. Here is a *shabu* recipe using *shoyu* and *tofu*, products of the chock-full-of-protein soybean to reinforce the fish protein.

Iso Shabu

2 quarts water
1 C dried bonito *(katsuobushi)*
2 C *sake*
3" square dried kelp *(konbu)*
⅔ C *shoyu*
⅓ C vinegar
1 Japanese white radish *(daikon)*
1 green pepper
3 green onions
　At least 3 kinds of fish or shellfish
　Seaweed, dried and soaked
8 large mushrooms, sliced
　Chinese cabbage, washed and sliced
½ cake *tofu*, sliced

Bring water to boil in an attractive pan or chafing dish. Add seaweed and bring back to boil. Remove seaweed. Stir in dried bonito and turn off heat. Add sake and the shoyu. Keep warm. Make a dipping sauce of the vinegar and an equal amount of shoyu. Grate radish and pepper and garnish with green onion. Place on small dishes in front of each guest. Arrange seafoods and vegetables cut in bite-sized chunks attractively on a large platter. Pass out the chopsticks and let each person have his turn at cooking whatever appeals to him in the hot broth. Fondue forks will do the trick if anyone balks at chopsticks. And don't forget to serve the broth.

Unsunaba Usachi

ENERGIZING SALAD. Many Hawaiian residents trace their roots to Okinawa in the Ryukyu Islands, south of their mother country Japan. Here is a *tofu*-Swiss chard salad, packed with energy.

1 bunch Swiss chard
½ block *tofu*
1 T honey
¼ C toasted sesame seeds
¼ t *shoyu*

*Wash chard. Cut up stems and steam. Add finely-
chopped leaves. Break tofu into pieces and boil 2 minutes. Drain. Grind the toasted seeds. Drain the tofu on
paper towels and squeeze out water. Mix with the seeds.
Add shoyu and honey. Fold in the Swiss chard and chill.
Serves three.*

Watercress with Tofu Sauce

WONDROUS LEAF. Watercress is a health food. The Japanese make
abundant use of it. Here are two recipes using watercress. The first is a
classic Japanese dish called *shira ae*.

1 bunch watercress
    Sauce:
2 t toasted sesame seeds
¼ cake *tofu*
3 T *miso*
1 T honey
½ t grated ginger

*In blender, blend sesame seeds until fine. Add tofu which
has been squeezed almost dry in a clean cloth. Add miso,
honey and ginger. Blend all together and pour over
watercress, which has been washed and boiled, excess
water removed and cut into 2-inch lengths. Place in serving dish.*

Wilted Sprouts and Watercress Salad

1 pkg. (12 ozs.) bean sprouts
1 bunch watercress, chopped

2 T sesame oil
2 T sesame seeds

Saute vegetables a couple of minutes in sesame oil and place in dish. Sprinkle sesame seeds over vegetables. Drizzle with tamari or soy sauce.

A few decades of race-mixing, food-mixing and culture-mixing results in new ways to enhance the taste and nutritional advantages of many foods.

UNUSUAL SOUP. Soups are popular in Hawai'i. Sometimes the tradewinds bring the temperatures down to the low 70's which feel like the 60's due to a wind chill factor, so soup is a welcome warmer-upper. *Saimin*, a Japanese noodle soup, is available on almost every street corner. But here is a soup using watercress instead of noodles.

Waikiki Watercress Soup

1   bunch watercress
1½ lbs. baking or red potatoes
½   C soy milk or dairy milk
1   sprig green onions, chopped
1½ C water

Wash watercress well. Pick off leaves and let drain in a colander. Cut tender stems into small pieces and blend, adding the 1½ cups of water a little at a time. Strain into a pitcher. Meanwhile, boil potatoes in 2¾ cups of water until tender. Blending a little at a time, whirl all ingredients except the milk. When dissolved, add milk. Consistency should be quite thick. Heat, adding more milk and butter to taste and a squeeze of lemon juice. Do not allow to boil. Serves 3.

A NUTRITIOUS JAPANESE SEA VEGETABLE

Some foods that are brimming with life energy are nevertheless overlooked by some peoples because of taste patterns. We call seaweed a weed because it is a nuisance. It interferes with the enjoyment of swimming and boating, and who would even dream of putting it into their mouth?

The Japanese would, and seaweed happens to be one of their best kept health secrets.

They call it a vegetable, not a weed. They put on high boots and wade into the ocean to harvest it.

You can do the same—if you know your seaweed. Be sure to pick out the bits of shell and wash it thoroughly. Then spread it out onto a paper towel to dry.

Or, you can buy it dried in the Oriental or gourmet sections of your supermarket. There are four popular types:

- *Nori* is said to be highest in minerals and protein. It comes in sheets which can be cut into strips and used as a garnish for soups and casseroles. Its flavor can be enhanced by roasting in a moderate oven 3 to 4 minutes before using.

- *Hijiki*, sometimes spelled *hiziki*, is high in calcium. The Japanese use it as a condiment that can be mixed with rice or used to flavor soybeans.

- *Konbu* contains certain amino acids that contribute to making complete proteins when used with other foods. The Japanese prize *konbu* for its subtle flavor and use it to attain the taste effects needed in certain of their dishes.

- *Kanten* is what we call *agar-agar*. It is a thickening agent used worldwide. The Japanese package it in double sticks that look like sliced-up sponge.

These four seaweeds will be discussed further here, but you are not limited to these types. The iodine, calcium and other valuable, easily absorbed minerals in this vegetable of the sea are found in whatever variety it grows.

When we lived on Long Island on the East Coast, we would often gather what we called "Irish Moss." High in vitamin A, it made an excellent thickening agent for stews or soups and could be substituted for *agar-agar* in any recipe, after soaking it for about a half-hour. You may have already tried *dulse*, which grows in abundance off both the East and West Coasts. High in calcium, it need not be soaked before use. It combines well with root vegetables. It can also be added to soups a few minutes before serving.

FOOD ADDITIVE. Getting back to *nori*, use the roasted bits in various ways to get used to the taste. Start with soup, then salad, then a fish dish. Experiment. Get to know it. It can be a lasting friend because it can contribute to your healthier, longer life. The Japanese eat *nori* straight, pickling or candying it.

Here is how to use *hijiki* as a condiment.

½ C dried *hijiki*
1 T oil
1 sliced onion
2 t *shoyu*
1 T vinegar

Wash and pick over hijiki. Soak about 10 minutes in water to cover. Cut into pieces and bring to boil for 5 minutes. Lower heat, cover and simmer 25 minutes. Meanwhile, saute onion and add to hijiki with the shoyu. Turn off heat, cover and leave on burner. When cool, add vinegar and refrigerate. It will keep one to two weeks.

SEA VEGETABLE DESSERT. Here are two ways to get the nutritional advantages of *kanten* in desserts. *Kanten* can be substituted for gelatin. It will mold even at room temperature and hold its shape for party dishes.

Kanten Dessert

2 sticks *kanten*
3½ C water or fruit juice
2 C sugar or 1 C honey
½ t lemon, vanilla or almond flavoring

Rinse kanten and squeeze dry. Shred into small pieces and soak in the 3½ cups of water for 30 minutes. Place on stove and heat until kanten melts. Add sugar and cook 10 to 15 minutes. Remove from heat, add flavoring and strain into an 8-inch square pan. Chill and cut into 1-inch squares.

Island Holidays Pudding

DESSERT WITHOUT SWEETENING. Here's a healthful dessert that calls for no sweetening of any kind. In addition to nutritious seaweed, it also uses that vital seed, sesame.

2   C apple juice
1   bar *kanten (agar-agar)*
6-8 T *tahini* (sesame seed paste)

Soak the kanten about 30 minutes. Squeeze out moisture. Heat about ½ cup of the apple juice. Shred in the kanten and boil until thoroughly dissolved. Stir in the remaining juice. Let mixture cool and thicken slightly. In a blender, blend together with the tahini. Chill and serve.

HOW TO USE JAPAN'S TOP PRIORITY HEALTH FOOD

JAPAN'S NO. 1 HEALTH FOOD. We have previously disclosed the food that heads the list of Japan's priority health foods: soybeans.

Three main products of the soybean are used daily in Japan: *shoyu, tofu* and *miso.*

Shoyu is a sauce obtainable in your supermarket. It is the same sauce that is usually found on the table in Chinese restaurants. Its chief ingredient is the soybean. We have already indicated its uses in recipes. You can extend its use in your home as far as your imagination and taste buds permit.

We will now discuss the preparation and use of *tofu* and *miso.* But, first, a word about using soybeans directly, as nature supplies them.

PROTEIN SNACK. If you can find green soybeans in the pod, steam them for about 15 minutes, let them cool and serve as a snack. It's fun to pop them open. They are so good plain that you really don't need a sauce to dip them into.

Dried soybeans should be soaked for several hours before cooking.

Change the water at least three times as the beans contain an anti-digestant enzyme that must be leached out before consuming.

After soaking, they can be cooked in a variety of ways, or you might like to sprout them instead. Soybean sprouts, whether purchased in plastic packages or sprouted at home, need to be parboiled before using.

Because of their high protein content, soybeans make an excellent meat substitute. You can make a soybean "meat loaf" by blending them, adding chopped onions, garlic, marjoram or oregano, and chopped green peppers. Season to taste. Pour a can of tomato soup over the loaf and top with cheese slices. Bake in a moderate oven for an hour.

Tofu, soybean curd, can now be made at home with special equipment. However, more and more supermarkets are stocking it as it grows in popularity in the U. S.

After you have purchased a cake of *tofu*, it should be removed from its plastic bag or container and washed gently. Now place it in a larger dish with a cover. The cake of *tofu* should be immersed in water which you must then change daily. This way you can use a little at a time and it will remain fresh in your refrigerator for about a week. If you wish to keep it a little longer, it should be steamed, simmered or fried for several minutes, and then re-covered with water and refrigerated.

Sliced *tofu* can be added to soups. Merely slice into bite-sized pieces and place in soup bowls. The hot soup will sufficiently heat it. Serve immediately.

Tofu can be blended in an electric blender and added to moulded dishes instead of cottage cheese or sour cream. This is a great boon to those who must eliminate dairy foods from their diets.

Here's a recipe that uses *tofu* and *soy* or *mung* sprouts in a delicious, meatless, though protein-rich dish.

Tofu and Sprouts Kokee

1 medium onion, sliced
1 clove garlic, chopped
1 slice of fresh ginger, chopped
1 cake of *tofu*
1 bag of sprouts
  butter or sesame oil
  shoyu to taste

Brown onion, garlic and ginger in butter or oil. Stir and add the sprouts. Cook for a few minutes, then add the tofu cut into squares. Drizzle with shoyu and serve. For 3-4.

Tofu is a great extender when scrambling eggs, or you can make:

Scrambled Tofu

½ cake *tofu*
1 egg
2 green onions, sliced
     dash of pepper, black or cayenne
1 T butter or sesame oil
1 t dried parsley
2 T *shoyu*

Rinse and drain tofu on paper towel. Saute onions and parsley in oil or butter. Break tofu into pieces and stir-fry in hot fat for several minutes. Add shoyu and seasonings and stir. Beat egg slightly and stir into mixture. Cook only until egg is firm. Serve immediately. Serves 2. Can be added to a clear broth.

Quick Beef-Tofu Bouillon

1 can beef bouillon
1 small clove garlic, minced
1 onion, chopped
¼ cake *tofu*, cubed
     Greens (optional)
1 t sesame oil
     Butter
1 tomato, chopped

Saute ginger, garlic and onion in small amount of butter. Add bouillon and can of water. Add tomatoes. Heat to simmer. Add tofu and greens that have been sliced fine for a couple of minutes only. Do not boil. Place ½ teaspoon oil in each bowl and add hot soup. Serves 2.

An easy way to add soy to your menu is to substitute instant soy powder (available in health food stores) to any recipe calling for powdered milk. It can also be used reconstituted in place of dairy milk. Stir carefully until smooth and use it freely, knowing you are giving a boost to your family's health.

Bean-threads or "long rice" are mistakenly thought to be made of soy. Actually, their basic ingredient is *mung* beans. To cook them, merely dip the fine threads into boiling water for about 10 minutes until tender. Drain and add flavoring, such as *shoyu*, leftover soup or gravy.

You have read about the benefits of *miso* in Chapter 6. You know now that it is the end product of a painstaking technique that renders soybean mash into a delectable delicacy that can be compared with European fine aged wines and cheeses.

It is most commonly used by the Japanese in soups. It will add new dimensions in flavoring your soups, if added just before serving. Be sure to stir until dissolved.

Basic Miso Soup

Scant cup of *iriko* (small dried fish)
10   T *miso*
5   C water
2½ T finely chopped green onions and
     tops
1⅔ C sliced *daikon* (turnip)

Wash iriko, add 5 cups of water and simmer for 15 minutes. Serves 6.

RECIPES FROM "THE LAND OF THE MORNING CALM"

The last of the three Asian countries to send workers into the Hawaiian fields was Korea, "Land of the Morning Calm." That was in 1903, and Koreans are still arriving today. They form a small but vital segment of Hawai'i's population.

Since they had emigrated from urban areas, they had already been exposed to Western ways and religious beliefs. They learned English quickly and adapted easily to island life. And they contributed their own secrets for the energy, vitality and love of life that they radiate.

As with other Eastern peoples, rice is the mainstay of the Korean diet. The Koreans like to offset its blandness at every meal with *kim-chee*, their unique contribution in the kaleidoscope of tastes in Hawai'i.

Our introduction to *kim-chee* came when we were tourists back in the early 1960's. We stopped in a market for some picnic food and picked up a package of some interesting looking chopped salad. Across the street, at Ala Moana Park, we sat in the shade of a *koa* tree and dug in. A passing Korean would have roared at our wry faces.

HEALTHFUL RELISH. This throat-searing relish is not meant to be eaten by itself. Whatever you eat it with is enhanced. Cabbage and apple cider vinegar, the vinegar we recommend that you use, are recognized health foods.

Here is the recipe for *kim-chee*, followed by several others from Korea.

Kim-Chee
(Paich'u Kimch'i)

1½-2 lbs. celery cabbage
3½ C water
1   C vinegar
¼ C sea salt
2   t finely chopped red pepper
1   T sugar
2   cloves garlic, finely chopped
¼ t finely chopped fresh ginger
½ small onion, thinly sliced

Wash cabbage and cut into 1½-inch lengths. Add salt to the vinegar and water and soak cabbage for four hours. Wash and drain it thoroughly. Add other ingredients and mix well. Press into a quart jar. Cover and refrigerate for several days to ripen. Serve as an accompaniment to a meat dish.

Korean Pupu Meatballs

POWER-PACKED SEED. In Hawaiian, the word *pupu* means shell but has come to mean an hors d'oeuvre. The power-packed seed is sesame.

1 pound ground round
1 block *tofu*
1 package (12 ozs.) bean sprouts
1 cup green onion, chopped fine
2 to 3 large cloves garlic, put through garlic press
¼ C roasted sesame seeds, ground or crushed
⅜ C plus 2 T soy sauce
2 T sugar
1 large egg
4 T sesame oil

*Dip bean sprouts into boiling water for about ½ minute.
Rinse in cold water. Chop into ½-inch lengths. Add to
ground beef. Squeeze water out of tofu using cheese
cloth. Mash and add to meat. Mix soy sauce and sugar
together before stirring into meat. Add remaining ingredients, mix well and shape into little balls. Brown in
heavy skillet in a little sesame oil.*

Watercress Salad
(Minali Namul)

Koreans recognize the health values of watercress, too.

1 bunch watercress
1 carrot, grated
1 t sesame oil
1 t toasted sesame seeds
¼ t sugar
⅛ t cayenne pepper
1 clove garlic, minced

*Wash watercress and cut into 1-inch lengths. Add carrots
if desired. Combine remaining ingredients and mix well.
Add sauce to watercress and carrots, mix and serve. 6
servings.*

Soybean Sprouts
(K'ong Nimul)

Nature lends a hand when you sprout your own. They come in cans, too.

1   lb. fresh soybean sprouts or
4   C canned bean sprouts
1½ t finely chopped green onions and tops
1   T sesame seeds, toasted
1   t *shoyu*
    dash cayenne pepper
1   T sesame oil

Wash and drain the fresh sprouts. Heat the oil and fry, stirring until done. Add the rest of the ingredients. If canned sprouts are used, just heat through, season and serve. 6 servings.

Long Rice with Vegetables
(Chop Chae)

This is one of our favorite Korean health dishes.

1 bundle long rice
2 dried mushrooms
¼ lb. beef
1 small carrot
1 thin stalk celery
1 small onion
¼ lb. green beans
½ can (15 ozs.) bamboo shoots
1 T sesame oil
1 T *shoyu*
2 t sugar
   salt and pepper to taste
⅛ C water

Soak long rice and mushrooms in warm water for half an hour. Cut beef into thin 2-inch strips. Remove stems from mushrooms. Cut mushroom caps and vegetables into thin strips or slices. Cut bundle of long rice in half and cook in 1 quart boiling water for 1 minute; drain thoroughly. In a large skillet, heat sesame oil. Fry beef for 1 minute. Add vegetables; saute 2 minutes. Combine shoyu, sugar, salt, pepper and ⅛ cup water. Stir long rice and shoyu mixture into vegetables; cook 2 minutes more. 3 servings.

Mountain Honey Wafers
(Yak Wa)

¾ C water
½ C brown sugar
1 T honey
1 T bourbon
3 C flour
⅓ C sesame oil
   deep fat for frying
1 C honey
⅛ C pine nuts, finely chopped
   Cinnamon

Combine water, brown sugar and 1 tablespoon honey. Bring to a boil; when cool, stir in bourbon. Mix flour and oil. Stir in syrup, making a stiff dough. On a floured board, roll dough ¼-inch thick; cut into 1-inch diamonds or squares. Heat deep fat to 400° F. Fry wafers until lightly browned; drain briefly on paper towels. Dip wafers in the cup of honey; drain in a colander. Roll in nuts and sprinkle with cinnamon. Store in a tightly covered container several days before serving. Makes 2½ dozen wafers.

FOOD WITH A FLAIR FROM THE PHILIPPINES

An influx of people to Hawai'i in the first decade of this century came from a land made up of 7000 islands which stretch from the Asian mainland south almost to Indonesia. Today, the Filipinos make up about 12 percent of the population of our state.

The dishes of the Philippines are as varied as its culture, which is basically Malayan-Indonesian with a sprinkle of Spanish, Chinese and American.

In the Philippines, each *barrio* or village has its own version of the national dishes which comprise the health-contributing proteins and minerals contained in fish, chicken, pork, seafoods, sweet potatoes (together with their leaves), sprouts, seaweed, beans, greens and rice.

FERMENTATION FOR LONGEVITY. They use pickled vegetables and fruits similar to their Korean and Japanese neighbors, and they include a fermented food, fermentation again providing that secret ingredient toward-longevity.

In the Philippines, this fermented food is called *bagoong* and it is used as a seasoning and an accompaniment for fish, meat and vegetables. It is made of small shrimp and fish, allowed to ferment, with salt added.

Watch the Philippine people in Hawai'i at one of their special celebrations, usually in June. As you admire their festive nature, their beauty, their joy in dance, music and games, you know they must be doing something right.

HIGH-PROTEIN FILIPINO DISHES. Here are some recipes brought to Hawai'i from the Philippines, using the foods that keep them perpetually in the prime of life.

Shrimp Sinigang

1 large lemon
1½ C sliced tomatoes
¾ C sliced onions
¾ lb. cleaned shrimps

⅓ C watercress, turnips or cabbage
Salt and pepper to taste

Squeeze lemon into 3 cups of water in a pot. Add to-matoes and onions and boil. Add shrimps and cook until pink. Chop vegetables and add to soup. Cook about one minute longer and serve.

Adobo with Chicken and Pork

Adobo is a Spanish-Filipino stew flavored with *shoyu* and spices. Simmer gently until the meat is tender.

 1¼ lbs. lean, boneless pork
 2 lbs. chicken legs and thighs
 ½ lb. liver
 ½ C each wine vinegar and water
 ¼ C *shoyu*
 8 whole black peppers
 1 bay leaf
 4 cloves garlic, minced or mashed
 2 T salad oil
  Chopped parsley
  Hot cooked rice

Cut pork into 1-inch cubes and combine with chicken and liver in a bowl. Pour in the vinegar, water and soy; add peppers, bay and garlic. Cover and refrigerate for about 1 hour, turning every now and then. Remove meats from marinade and pat dry saving the marinade. Heat the oil in a Dutch oven (don't use a cast-iron pan) over medium high heat. Cook the liver until brown and just firm, about 3 minutes; remove from pan. Put in chicken and brown all over; remove from pan. Put in pork and cook, stirring until browned. Pour in reserved marinade, cover and simmer pork for 15 minutes. Return the chicken to pan, cover and simmer for 30 minutes longer. Remove to serving platter to keep warm while remaining liquid is boiled until condensed. 6 servings.

Noodles with Pork and Shrimp
(Pansit)

1   pkg. (8 ozs.) fine egg noodles
1   lb. pork
½   lb. shrimp
1   T salad oil
1   clove garlic, crushed
1   small onion, sliced
     dash of pepper
2   T *shoyu*

Cook noodles in boiling salted water until tender; drain thoroughly. Cut pork into small pieces. Shell and clean shrimp. In a large skillet, heat oil. Saute garlic briefly, then remove. Add onion and saute lightly. Stir in pork and cook until pork is lightly browned. Add shrimp and seasonings and saute until pork and shrimp are thoroughly cooked. Stir in shoyu and cooked noodles. Garnish with chopped peanuts, chopped bacon, lemon slices and finely chopped green onions. 6 servings.

Coconut Dessert
(Bucayo)

4   C shredded coconut
½   C water
2   C sugar
½   t anise or vanilla flavoring

Combine water and sugar and boil to 236 degrees until the syrup forms a soft ball in cold water. Add the coconut and cook slowly for 20 minutes until the coconut is transparent. Cool, add the flavoring and serve chilled. Serves 8.

Sans Rival

This is a rich layered dessert from the Philippines. Fruits can be substituted for the nuts.

6   eggs, separated
¾   C sugar
¼   C water
1   C sugar
1   bar of butter
2   T rum
⅓   C nut bits, such as macadamia, walnut or cashew

Beat the whites of eggs with ¾ cup of sugar into a meringue. Let stand. Now boil the water with 1 cup of sugar until syrupy. Cut the butter in and stir until melted. Remove from heat and pour a little at a time over the egg yolks which have been beaten together, alternating with the rum. Spread the meringue on well-greased cookie sheets (you'll need 4) and cook about 20 minutes at 350 degrees. Remove before it browns. Let cool. Spread the meringue sheets with the filling and sprinkle with the nuts, one on top of the other. It should form a loaf. Wrap in wax paper or foil and freeze. Cut just before serving.

WESTERN INFLUENCES IN HAWAI'I

People who arrived in Hawai'i to work in the sugar cane and pineapple fields were not only from the Pacific. It is just 100 years since the Portuguese came from the island of Madeira in the Azores. Perhaps their healthful influence preceded them, because long before this, Portuguese seamen had introduced maize, rice, oranges, tobacco and the sweet potato into many lands. Virile and health-minded, they brought *"materia medica"* from their homeland to Asian ports.

China is indebted to these intrepid voyagers for introducing pineapple, papaya, guava and watercress. To this day, they call watercress the Portuguese vegetable *(Sai Yeung Choi)* and value it nutritionally as a food and medically as a diuretic.

To Hawai'i, the Portuguese brought the *ukulele,* the guitar and the *taro*-patch fiddle, all of which played important parts in the development of modern Hawaiian music.

Their ethnic dishes that are common in Hawai'i today include spicy Portuguese sausage, sweet bread, bean soup and naughty fried and sugary doughnuts called *malassadas*.

For a healthy taste of Madeira, try this chicken dish.

Chicken Apritada

2	lbs. chicken, cut into serving-sized pieces
2	cloves garlic, crushed
¼	C oil
	salt and pepper to taste
1	small can sliced pimento
1	can garbanzo beans
2	potatoes, peeled and quartered
1	can tomato sauce
½	C water
1	t *shoyu*
1	bay leaf
1	t sugar

Brown chicken in oil with garlic. Season with salt and pepper. When browned, add pimento, garbanzo beans, potatoes, tomato sauce, water, shoyu, sugar and bay leaf. Cover and cook until potatoes are tender. Serves 4.

Portuguese Bean Soup

INEXPENSIVE NUTRITION. The following is an island favorite that packs a lot of nutrition into a budget meal.

1¼	C dried navy beans or
16	ozs. kidney beans
¾	lb. smoked ham or
2	ham hocks
2	potatoes, pared and cubed
2	carrots, sliced

    2   onions, chopped
    1   small cabbage, chopped
    2   celery stalks, chopped
    2   garlic cloves, minced
    2   sprigs of parsley, minced
    2   bay leaves
          salt and pepper to taste
    ½   t Dijon mustard
    2   C tomato sauce
    8   C water

Dry beans should be soaked overnight. Bring water to boil and simmer ham for an hour. Add beans. Then add all other ingredients except sausage and cook for 2 hours. Now add the sausage and simmer for 1 hour more.

Another island in the Atlantic that made its Pacific contribution is Puerto Rico. Its people brought with them the Spanish influence and their *cocina criolla*, a good ambassador for the Creole cuisine of the Caribbean.

For seasonings, the Caribbean cuisine makes use of lime-rind, cinnamon, cloves, pepper, fresh ginger, garlic and sour oranges. Oregano and coriander (Chinese parsley) are favored herbs.

They make a coconut pudding which is identical to Hawaiian *haupia*, with the addition of a tablespoon of orange blossom water. Here are two Puerto Rican recipes that have become "rooted" in Hawai'i.

Sancocho

BALANCED ENERGY BOOSTER. This is a stew of vegetables and meat.

    1   lb. stewing beef
    ¼   lb. cubed pork
    1   large tomato
    1   large onion
    1-2   cloves garlic
    1   green pepper

1¾ C water
4   ozs. tomato sauce
1   C pumpkin
1   C yams
1   C potatoes
1   C *taro* (optional)
     salt and pepper to taste

Combine meat and chopped tomatoes, onion, green pepper and garlic cloves with the water. When brought to a boil, turn down heat and simmer about 1 hour. Now stir in the tomato sauce and cubed vegetables. Continue to simmer until they are tender. Serves 5.

Arroz Con Pollo

This is a rice and chicken dish with a Spanish flavor.

2¾ lbs. chicken pieces
1   t oregano
2   peppercorns
1   clove garlic
2   t salt
2   t olive oil
1   t vinegar
1   T oil
3   T *sofrito*
6   pitted green olives
1   t capers
1   tomato
2   T oil or *achiote* lard
½   t paprika
2   ozs. ketchup
2   C rice, washed and drained
1   pkg. frozen peas
2¾ C water
1   4-oz. can pimentos

Mash oregano, pepper, garlic, salt and olive oil in a

mortar and rub into chicken pieces. Heat 1 tablespoon of oil and brown chicken lightly. Add 3 tablespoons prepared sofrito *(see below). Reduce heat. Add chopped olives, tomato and capers. Cook 10 minutes. Add the 2 tablespoons of oil and paprika and rice and cook 5 more minutes. Add water, mix well and cook on high flame uncovered until dry. Stir up rice from bottom. Cover and simmer for about 20 minutes more. Add peas, turn rice again, cover and cook for 10 minutes more. Garnish dish with pimentos. Serves 4-5.*

Sofrito

¼ C vegetable oil
½ lb. green peppers, chopped
⅛ lb. sweet chili peppers
½ lb. onions, chopped
6 cloves garlic, peeled
8 coriander leaves
1 T oregano
¼ lb. cured ham, chopped
½ C vegetable oil

Whirl all ingredients but the last two at high speed in a blender. Now add the ham and blend all together. Heat remaining oil and add the crushed ingredients. Bring to boil, lower heat and cook 15 minutes. Place in glass jar, cover and refrigerate. Will keep for several weeks.

THE NEWEST ARRIVALS IN HAWAI'I

The mixture of cultures continues. And maybe the mixture is part of the health picture, a new dimension to the concept of the balanced diet.

The latest arrivals are the Vietnamese. Among the first jobs they take are as cooks and chefs, so Vietnamese items are beginning to appear on Hawaiian menus.

An example is this tasty one-dish meal.

Dark and Crusty Chicken

Chicken legs (10-12)
Sesame oil
Freshly ground black pepper
Cinnamon
Orange juice
Ketchup
shoyu
1 small Chinese mustard cabbage
1 small green pepper
8 cherry tomatoes
2 sprigs parsley
2 zucchinis, sliced
1 package noodles
butter

Remove skin from chicken parts. Place in oven pan, sprinkle with pepper and cinnamon and dot with oil. Pour orange juice over chicken ¼ inch deep. Broil at 350 degrees for 15 minutes. Now cover with ketchup and let it drip down into the pan. Stir into juices and cook about 10 more minutes. Turn over, sprinkle with more cinnamon and cook 12 minutes more. If the chicken begins to char, turn down the heat. Boil noodles until just done. Drain and add butter to pan. Cut vegetables in chunks. Stir-fry in butter mixed with a little sesame oil until wilted in a wok or large skillet. Add tomatoes. Cover and turn off heat. Place noodles on center of chop plate, cover with chicken, and pour sauce over it. Arrange vegetables and garnish with parsley. Serves 4.

12

Tips for Parties and Games That Capture Island Vitality

In this chapter, we let our hair down and have some fun. Fun is therapeutic. The Hawaiians are the happiest people on earth and this can be one reason why they are the healthiest. You can hold a *lu'au*, imbue your home or apartment with the feeling of Hawai'i, and try out some of the Hawaiian games of strength and skill.

You will learn of:

LONGEVITY FACTOR

CHEMICAL-FREE BEER

RUM DRINK WITH FRUIT

THERAPEUTIC CLOTHES

THE THERAPY OF FLOWERS

THERAPEUTIC WORDS

TUNE IN TO MUSIC

NO. 1 HAWAIIAN HEALTH SECRET

TIME AS A HEALTH FACTOR

LONGEVITY FACTOR. Laughter is therapeutic. Fun and joy are the best medicines. Island people appear to have known this all along. The rest of us are just beginning to discover the incredible effectiveness of laughter in restoring health and prolonging life.

When Norman Cousins of the *Saturday Review of Literature* was seriously ill and given a poor prognosis by his doctors, he checked out of the hospital and into a hotel where he read humorous books and magazines and played laughing records to trigger his own guffaws. He was soon cured, much to the surprise of the medical community.

Cousins knew what the Pacific islanders know. Laughter is good for whatever ails you and it is a good preventive for ailments.

Hawaiians and Tahitians are, in our opinion, the best examples of joyous people. The fun-loving Hawaiians have become known worldwide for their lilting music, their hula dancing and their festive *lu'aus*.

We can all gain in health and vitality by closing some doors to stressful matters and opening other doors to fun and frivolity.

Islanders hold no monopoly on lighthearted living, but they do give us good examples to emulate. The *lu'au* is perhaps the best.

Early *lu'aus* in Hawai'i were called *'aha 'aina*, or feast gatherings. On the menu might be *taro, taro* tops, *poi*, breadfruit, sweet potato, yam, banana, seaweed, fish and chicken—all surrounding a whole pig or dog, steamed in an underground oven. (Don't eye Rover or Spot as a possible main course, because the ancient Hawaiians used a special breed of vegetable-fed dog that was more like wild game than domestic canine.)

There was music, dance, chanting and singing, all of which—including the eating and drinking—went on for many hours.

Today, it is still the same—except for the dog! It is not unusual for 1000 people to attend a *lu'au*. But *lu'aus* that are held under the palm trees in natural settings are getting rarer. If the palm trees are there, so are nearby hotels. There are *lu'aus* sponsored by the hotels for visitors, *lu'aus* sponsored by churches to raise funds, and *lu'aus* sponsored by organizations to commemorate events. There are private *lu'aus* to celebrate a baby's first birthday and other occasions.

We have attended *lu'aus* on a pier, in a convention hall and in a school.

The important ingredient is letting go of anxieties, diets, restraints and hang-ups—and letting in relaxation and release.

HOW TO HAVE YOUR OWN LU'AU

If you want to be the talk of the town, hold a *lu'au*.

We held one when we lived on another island—Long Island, New York. We had the help of a Hawaiian *wahini* (woman) who lived nearby and danced at a Polynesian restaurant. She provided the authentic entertainment as well as many ideas and decorations.

We named the punchbowl "Punchbowl," which is where, coincidentally, we happen to now live on O'ahu. We filled our water cooler (we knew enough to drink bottled spring water in that area) with *mai tais*, one of the most powerful of drinks, and it appeared to play a major role in making that *lu'au* an "historical" event.

But you do not need a Hawaiian hula dancer or a water cooler full of *mai tais*. "Do your own thing."

Plan ahead. Here are some main areas to start thinking about:

1. Decor
2. Table setting
3. *Leis*
4. Music and entertainment
5. Where to get help
6. Menu

Let's take these one at a time. For decor, if the weather is mild, a garden or patio is perfect. If you live in an apartment, see if you can get the use of the common recreational facilities for that afternoon or evening. You can transform your indoors into a tropical setting with house plants and flowers.

Candles are tropical. So are flaming *tiki* torches, if you are outside. Put pineapples and coconuts on the tables and in corner niches.

As for your table, use a green cloth or get a paper one printed with a *tapa* design. Consider bamboo mats or even woven beach mats.

As your centerpiece, pile up pineapples, coconuts, papayas and bananas. Or use a striking piece of coral if you have one. How about a fishnet cloth with a primitive sculpture set on ferns in the center? Express your own feelings as you set the stage for feast and fiesta Hawaiian style.

Flowers are therapeutic. In England, essences of flowers are used as remedies for depression, nervousness and other mental ailments. In Hawai'i, the flowers themselves say, "Look at me and forget your problems."

A necklace of flowers, called a *lei*, can be strung like beads. You can make a *lei* of daisies, dandelions, carnations or whatever flowers are available. At our Long Island *lu'au*, we were surrounded by rhododendrons, so we strung them on nylon fishing line. But crochet thread will do as well. If you cannot obtain fresh flowers, try for plastic *leis* at your party goods store, or have the children make bright crepe paper "blossoms," and then spray them with a flowery cologne. Check with your florist for ideas.

Leis may seem to pose a problem. But it is a problem worth solving. There is nothing like putting a flower *lei* around an arriving guest's neck,

along with the traditional accompanying kiss, to get a party started on a
high level of gaiety.

As for entertainment, a *ukulele* or a guitar is the key. If you know
someone who plays either, collar him. Maybe there are Hawaiians living
in your city or town. They are always happy to share their *aloha* and their
culture with those who are sincerely interested.

If you live near New York, Chicago, Los Angeles, San Francisco, or
Washington, D. C., contact the Hawai'i Visitors Bureau which has offices
in those cities. They can help you locate Hawaiian caterers or entertainers, and possibly recommend shops that stock Hawaiian decorations.

How about putting up some Hawaiian posters for decorations? Here
your local travel agency can be of help. Check with your library for short
films on Hawai'i that you might show and, while you are there, check out
some Hawaiian words you can sling around at the *lu'au*, such as:

- *"Aloha no"*   (welcoming guests at the door)
- *"Mahalo"*   (thank you)
- *"Komo mai e'ai"*   (announcing dinner)
- *"Ono"*   (delicious)
- *"Hana hou!"*   (encore!)

HEALTHFUL HAWAIIAN DISHES FOR A MEMORABLE LU'AU

Now for your *lu'au* menu.

At a modern, yet still authentic *lu'au* in Hawai'i, you would likely be
served shellfish and seaweed to start, followed by steamed crabs. Then
there would be fish baked in *ti* leaves and chicken cooked with *taro* tops
in coconut milk, accompanied by baked sweet potatoes and *poi*.

Then would come the *kalua* pig which has been baking in an underground oven all day. There would also be *lomi* salmon (salmon minced
with tomatoes), *haupia* (coconut pudding), and fresh fruit, especially
pineapple and banana.

Recipes for baked fish, *lomi* salmon and *haupia* are in Chapter 10.
As for the *kalua* pig, chances are you won't be able to build an underground oven for this one occasion. So consider roasting a whole suckling
pig in your oven, or a large ham or pork butt. Wrap it in foil in lieu of
leaves.

If you buy the dehydrated *poi* and reconstitute it according to the directions on the jar, serve only small portions. It will not bring raves from your guests, as one must really develop a taste for it. Still, it is a conversation piece and, if it is absent, you will not have a real *lu'au*.

On the other hand, no other dish mentioned is a must. If you have the *poi* and the pork, you have the backbone of the *lu'au*. The rest of the menu can be Oriental, Indian or just tropical. It will still be *lu'au*.

Take one feast, add a dash of merriment, and you have a *lu'au*. Its healthful aspect is the fun and laughter, the release from the cares of the day and freedom from stress.

You can make your guests forget themselves and act naturally with an atmosphere of festivity and "anything goes." The food sets the climate for this release. So the food must itself be a release from the conventional. Here are some unconventional entrees that fit well into a *lu'au*.

Hawaiian Curried Chicken

This can take the place of chicken cooked with *taro* tops, which are not available on the U. S. mainland. Not long after Captain Cook arrived two centuries ago, curry was introduced to the islands and was quickly accepted. This chicken curry dish takes about 1½ hours to prepare. It can be done the day before, refrigerated and then reheated. It serves 8.

5-6 lbs. chicken parts
1½ C water
3   ozs. bacon fat
3   medium onions, finely chopped
1   garlic clove
1   t powdered ginger
3   T ginger juice (from preserved ginger)
2   T finely chopped bacon cooked dry
2   T curry powder
    salt and pepper to taste
2   C chicken stock (from cooked chicken)
1   12-oz. can coconut milk
2   C brown rice, cooked

Cook bacon until dry. Remove and drain. Brown chicken

*parts in bacon fat until golden. Remove to deep pot,
cover with water and simmer until tender. Reserve
liquid.*

*In remaining bacon fat (add a little salad oil if neces-
sary), saute onions and garlic until transparent. Add
ginger, ginger juice, the chopped, cooked bacon, the
curry powder, salt and pepper. Now add the stock from
the cooked chicken and let it come to a boil. Add the
coconut milk and stir. Turn off heat. Pour over the
cooked chicken and refrigerate until serving time. Heat
slowly but do not overcook. Serve with fluffy brown rice
and the following in individual bowls: chutney, grated
coconut, chopped macadamia or almonds, finely
chopped hard-boiled eggs, raisins, chopped green onions, additional crumbled, dried, cooked bacon.*

Chicken and Spinach in Coconut Milk

Here is another chicken dish that is authentically Hawaiian and, in
fact, comes even closer to the chicken served at a Hawaiian *lu'au*, using
spinach instead of *taro* leaves.

1 lb. chicken, cut up
2 lbs. spinach (frozen or fresh)
¼ t salt
3 T melted butter
   boiling water
1 can coconut milk or
1 C shredded packaged coconut
½ C milk

*Fry chicken pieces in butter until brown. Add salt and
pour boiling water over chicken and simmer until tender.
If fresh spinach is used, wash thoroughly and cook.
Drain and chop or put in blender. If coconut milk is
unavailable, combine dried coconut and milk and soak
15 minutes. Simmer for 10 minutes more. Place in several thicknesses of cheesecloth and squeeze out all of the*

liquid. Drain the chicken. Add the spinach and coconut milk. Simmer 5 minutes and serve at once. 6 servings.

Hukilau Fish

The Chinese influence in Hawai'i gives you every right to serve this fish dish garnished with sesame seeds.

- 4   lbs. fish
- 1⅓ C water
- ⅔   C *shoyu*
- 3   slices fresh ginger root
- 3   garlic cloves
- 1⅓ C water
- ¼   C honey
       Garnish: sesame seeds, chopped green onions and parsley
       Cooked noodles

Steam fish for 20 minutes. (You can devise a steamer by placing fish on a rack set in your oven broiler pan. Cover with foil and cook over top burner.) Mix together all ingredients but the garnish and heat to below boiling point. When fish is tender and translucent, place on top of noodles on a large serving plate. Add some of the liquid from the steamer to the sauce and pour over the fish. Garnish with green onions and parsley and sprinkle with sesame seeds. Serves 6.

SERVE PUPUS INSTEAD OF HORS D'OEUVRES

Before your meal begins, when the beer, punch and *mai tais* are flowing, you will want to serve Hawaiian-style hors d'oeuvres, or *pupus*.

One of our favorites is influenced by the Japanese. Mash a hard-cooked egg with a little mayonnaise and ½ teaspoon of *miso*. We spread it on slices of cooked lotus root. But it is just as delicious on cucumber slices or crackers.

Here are three more *pupus* your *lu'au* guests will enjoy.

Stuffed Lychees

One that appears at the nicest parties is delicious and yet simple to prepare. Canned lychees are stuffed with cream cheese. Place on a platter and garnish with parsley, stuffed olives, strips of pimento or fresh flowers.

Pineapple Banana Pupu

    small bamboo skewers
2 cans sterno
1 fresh pineapple
3 firm bananas
1 C rum
1 C sugar

Cut pineapple into chunks. Cut each banana into 4 parts. Sprinkle with lemon juice to prevent darkening. Arrange bowls of rum and sugar for dipping. Have guests put fruit chunks on skewers and glaze over sterno or charcoal.

Teriyaki Sauce

1 t ginger powder or
2-inch piece fresh ginger root
2 garlic cloves
4 T ketchup
1 C *shoyu*
½ C honey
3 ozs. *sake* or sherry
    dash of Worcestershire sauce
4 T water

Mince together garlic and ginger. Place in pan with other ingredients and simmer, stirring for about 25 minutes. Refrigerate in covered jar until ready to use. Use over shrimps, small meatballs or raw fish.

SPECIAL SALADS FOR A LUʻAU

Salads do not have to be commonplace. It would be a mistake to serve the usual lettuce salad at a *luʻau*. A fruit salad makes more Polynesian sense. A tropical fruit salad is still better.

Here is a recipe for a special *luʻau* fruit salad:

Halakea Salad

1 large pineapple (cut as in pineapple banana *pupu*)
1 pt. strawberries
2 navel oranges
1 small, ripe avocado
½ C mayonnaise
½ C yogurt (fruit-flavored)

Place bite-sized pineapple pieces in a large bowl. Hull, wash and halve the berries. Pare and section one of the oranges. Slice avocado and add all fruits to the bowl. From the remaining orange, squeeze 2 tablespoons of juice, grate 1 teaspoon rind and stir into the blended mayonnaise and yogurt. Stand pineapple shell on platter. Fill with fruit mixture. Serve with dressing in separate bowl.

Papaya Seed Dressing

If you must serve greens or standard mainland fruits, then at least use a tropical dressing like this one.

¾ C honey
1 C cider vinegar
   dash of salt
1 t dry mustard
1 C sesame or olive oil
1 small, finely-chopped onion
3 T fresh papaya seeds

*In a blender, place honey, salt, mustard and vinegar.
Turn on blender and gradually add the cup of oil and
onions. Add seeds and blend to consistency of coarsely
ground pepper. Equally good over fruit or greens.*

Cucumber Salad

A Japanese salad still has a taste of Hawai'i. This one uses easy-to-
obtain ingredients.

3   C sliced cucumber, peeled
1   T coarse salt
1   C water
2   T vinegar
1   T *shoyu*
2   t sesame seeds
      dash cayenne pepper
1-2 cloves garlic
2   T green onions
½   t sugar

*Slice cucumber thin. Sprinkle with salt and add water.
Soak for 15 minutes. Drain off liquid. Add other ingredients, mix and chill at least 1 hour. 6 servings.*

EASY-TO-MAKE LUʻAU DESSERTS

A *luʻau* has to be fun for the hosts, too. Spread the preparation over a
number of days so that you are not too tired to enjoy your own party. Here
are some easy-to-make Hawaiian-type desserts that will top off your *luʻau*
feast with a proper flourish.

Macadamia Topped Banana Split

*Slice ripe bananas in half and spread with nut butter or
tahini. Sprinkle with broken bits of macadamia nuts.*

Avocado Rum Macadamia Chiffon Pie

This delectable dessert is served at the Hotel Hana-Maui.

Baked 9″ pie crust
1 C mashed ripe avocado
4 egg yolks
1 T butter
2 T sugar
    dash cinnamon and nutmeg
    juice of ½ lemon
1 T gelatin
4 T rum
4 egg whites
½ C sugar
4 T macadamia nuts
whipped cream

In a pan, cook together the avocado, egg yolks, butter, spices, lemon juice and sugar. Soften gelatin in the rum and add to hot mixture. Stir until dissolved. Cool in refrigerator. Beat egg whites until stiff with the remaining sugar. Fold into gelatin mixture. Pour into cooled baked pie shell. Decorate with whipped cream and sprinkle with the macadamia nuts.

Macadamia Nut Cookies

½ lb. butter
¼ C honey
1 t almond flavoring
dash of salt
½ pt. chopped macadamia nuts
2 C whole wheat flour

Cream honey and butter. Add flavoring, salt and nuts

and stir together. Now add flour a little at a time, stir-
ring. Roll dough into small balls. Bake on ungreased
cookie sheet for 15 minutes at 350 degrees. Do not let
brown. 4 dozen.

Jade Pudding

This is a very rich "quickie." In a blender place one
peeled, very ripe avocado and the juice of two small
limes or one medium lemon. Add about 3-4 tablespoons
of honey and blend all together. Pour into stemmed
glasses. Serves three.

Tropical Cheese Pie

Made with bananas, pineapple and *tofu* "cheese," this is a high-
protein dessert. Use two 9-inch pie pans.

> 1 block of *tofu*, drained
> 3 eggs
> ⅓ C honey
>   Juice of 1 lime
> 2 t grated lime peel
> 1 t vanilla
> 1 t orange liqueur
> 2 large ripe bananas
> 1 8½-oz. can crushed pineapple

In a blender combine eggs, honey, lime juice and flavor-
ings. Whirl for a moment. Now break up tofu and banana
into chunks. Add half to blender and whirl until smooth.
Add rest and blend again. Stir in pineapple (do not blend
again) and pour mixture into two cooked and cooled
graham cracker shells. (We substitute wheat germ,
sesame and sunflower seed meal for ¼ of the graham
crackers.) Bake at 325 degrees for an hour until
browned. Refrigerate. Can be decorated with sliced
strawberries and topped with whipped cream if desired.

FOUR PARTY DRINKS POLYNESIANS HAVE MADE FAMOUS

We have mentioned the ancient Polynesian drink *'awa*, or *kawa,* used in traditional ceremonies. It is still a special occasion drink on some of the islands of Polynesia.

But today in Hawai'i, wines and liquors are imported from all over the world. The Hawaiian liquor store looks just like yours.

Still, the Hawaiians tend to drink healthier party drinks than most mainlanders. That is because their mixers are not the carbonated kind, but rather fruit juices, milk and coconut milk.

We still have our *'okolehao*, originally a liquor distilled from the *ti* root, which has evolved into a sort of gin that can be made from either rice or pineapple juice. Pineapple juice is also made into a wine on the island of Maui.

CHEMICAL-FREE BEER. Primo beer, when it was made in Hawai'i, was one of only three made in the United States today without the use of chemicals. Add to this important quality the fact that it was made with pure water and you get a beer that is healthier to drink than any other. However, efforts to market Primo beer in mainland cities has not proved successful at this writing. It is now being made on the mainland.

Hawai'i also boasts a company that brews *sake*, a Japanese rice wine. But, surprisingly, we do not have any company making rum, which one usually finds in a sugar-growing area.

RUM DRINK WITH FRUIT. The most famous Hawaiian drink is a modern invention which we have already mentioned—made with rum— the *mai tai*.

Mai Tai

4 ozs. light rum
4 ozs. dark rum
2 ozs. lemon or lime juice
2 ozs. pineapple juice
2 ozs. brandy
1 oz. Triple Sec
crushed ice

Fill glasses ⅓ with crushed ice. Pour in mixed ingredients and top with more dark rum. Garnish with a slice of pineapple, a sprig of mint and a flower. (Here we use Vanda orchids.) Serves 4.

Here is an island recipe for punch and one for egg nog. The latter you might wish to save for the morning after your *lu'au*.

Paniolo Punch

    4 ozs. light rum
    1 C lime juice
    1 C guava juice (canned)
    ½ C pineapple juice (canned)
    1 C crushed ice

Place all ingredients in a blender and whirl for ½ minute until frothy. Pour into chilled glasses and serve. 4 servings.

Island Egg Nog

Take your favorite recipe for egg nog and substitute coconut milk for the cream. You'll love it and so will your guests.

Chi-Chi

Finally, the famous *Chi-Chi*, fast becoming appreciated for its mild "high."

    3 ozs. vodka
    3 ozs. Triple Sec
    4 ozs. coconut milk
    3 ozs. sweet/sour lemon mix
    3 ozs. pineapple juice
    crushed ice

Mix ingredients together. Pour into glass over crushed ice. Serves 2.

HOW TO BRING THE FEELING OF HAWAI'I
INTO YOUR HOME

If you cannot travel the thousands of miles to Hawai'i, you can bring a piece of Hawai'i into your home.

There was a company formed some years ago that canned Hawaiian air. The cans sold so well in department stores all over the United States that the company could not keep up with the orders and folded.

You certainly will not benefit by sniffing canned air, even if it comes from Hawai'i. But if there are other things you can do to capture the feeling of Hawai'i in your home, you will most certainly benefit from them.

Suppose you had a choice of artwork to hang on your walls. Which of these two categories would appeal to you most: city scenes with traffic, smog and maybe a street fight in progress, or country scenes with mountains, streams and maybe some cattle grazing or birds in flight?

We hope you selected the second category. Nature's tapestries contribute to health by counteracting stress.

Suppose you had a choice of music and you needed to play some music now as a way to revive your spirits. Which of these two categories would you select: hard rock, or soft melodies?

Again, we hope you selected the second category. Hard rock adds to the level of stress. Softer music is quieting and relaxing.

Hawaiian scenes for your artwork and Hawaiian songs for your music multiply the beneficial effects of passive scenes and melodious music. This is because Hawai'i is the symbol of the peace and joy that we all seek. It is a double—even triple—dose of good "medicine."

There are many other ways you can take this good "medicine":

- Prepare Hawaiian-type dishes
- Wear Hawaiian-type clothes
- Use Hawaiian words
- Read about Hawai'i

We have already provided you with recipes you can use. But even keeping a whole fresh pineapple in sight, with leafy tops intact, you will reap the benefit of a therapeutic sight.

How can sights be therapeutic? Which would you rather look at on your dining room table: golden pineapples and papayas, or canned peaches?

THERAPEUTIC CLOTHES. The clothes you wear can provide the same feeling When a man puts on a crazy tropical straw hat while weeding the lawn, he feels the rigors of office life fade into the background and disappear.

When a woman puts on a colorful *mu'umu'u* with a label on it that reads "Made in Hawai'i," she is free of the drudgery that binds her, and all the cells of her body, in effect, do a hula.

THE THERAPY OF FLOWERS. Think flowers. Put one in your hair. Keep some in the house whenever the price is right. Grow them. Admire their beauty. Permit their fragrance to take you to a magical isle.

THERAPEUTIC WORDS. Instead of saying "hello" or "goodbye," say *"aloha."* Feel the love of humanity carry away all the competitiveness and insecurity that may be tightening your muscles and causing stress.

"Aloha" feels so good to say in Hawai'i. But let it be said in your home, too. Let it bring love and affection.

Say *"mahalo"* instead of "thank you." Say *"ono ono"* instead of "delicious." Sound is vibration. These words have "good vibes."

You can call each other by your Hawaiian name equivalents (George is Keoki, Susan is Suke, Mary is Malia, John is Keoni). A good mainland source for further information on the Hawaiian language is Orchids of Hawai'i International, Inc., 305 Seventh Avenue, New York, New York 10001. For $1.00 they will send you a guide listing both common words and name translations.

Books about Hawai'i and record albums of Hawaiian music can be better medicines than the aspirin in your medicine cabinet.

Look in the travel section of your book store for books about Hawai'i. If a novel is published with a Hawaiian theme, read it. Children will have fun reading paperbacks published about life in Hawai'i by the Polynesian Voyaging Society.* These are the people who planned and executed that

---

*1355 Kalihi Street, Honolulu, Hawaii 96819.

momentous voyage to Tahiti, in the ancient way, as part of the Bicentennial celebration.

TUNE IN TO MUSIC. Your record shop carries many albums by Hawaiian entertainers. Ask about the one put out by the National Geographic Society. It has excellent background material on the history of island music.

Listen to music by Emma Veary, Palani Vaughn, George Helm, Ed Kenny, the Beamers, or the Brothers Cazimero. Maybe Cecilio and Kapono are more to your liking. Songs run the gamut from "golden oldies" to a more modern beat. It's a whole new world of music with steel guitars, nose flutes and *pahu*, the Polynesian drums. Tune in!

HAWAIIAN GAMES TO INCREASE
STRENGTH AND SKILL

Some of the games that Hawaiian youngsters and their families play today were popular a thousand years ago. There was a four-month period in autumn called *Makahiki*, when Hawaiians enjoyed freedom from everyday labors and oppressive obligations. It was celebrated with games and sports tournaments.

There were boxing and wrestling matches, surfing and diving competitions, canoe racing, tug-of-war, and *ti* leaf sliding down mud banks. Chiefs raced their land sleds down prepared courses on hilly terrain.

Many modern games that are played around the world today had their origins or counterparts in Hawai'i. There is evidence for this in such games as hide-and-seek, kite flying, stilt-walking, cat's cradles (these string games were formerly accompanied by chants), top-spinning and jacks.

NO. 1 HAWAIIAN HEALTH SECRET. Hawaiians like their fun and games. Their brimming good health has to be due at least in part to their fun-loving nature. In fact, we would call the top Hawaiian health secret not the food, not the fresh air, not the ocean, but the carefree life style that acts as a buffer to any stress that civilization tries to lay on them.

This fun-loving, carefree attitude makes the Hawaiians receptive to games of strength and skill. Here are a few typically Hawaiian games that you might like to try:

Hakoko
(Hawaiian Wrestling)

Face your opponent. At a mutual signal, try to obtain a wrestling hold. The object is to force your opponent to the ground. When any part of him, except the soles of his feet, touches the ground, you score a point.

Hakoko Noho
(Seated Wrestling)

This is done by opponents seated on grass or mats facing each other with right legs extended in front and left feet tucked under right knees. Sit close together so you can reach each other. Left hands go on each other's right shoulders. Right hands go on each other's waists. The bent left knees should be in contact. Now try to topple your opponent, unseating him by pushing him over sideways with your right hand, aided by your left. The first one who releases one hand to break or prevent a fall loses.

Pa Uma
(Wrist Wrestling)

Stand facing your opponent with your right foot toe-to-toe with his right foot. Clasp right hands so that each is grasping the other's right thumb. Without moving feet, try to push his hand back so you touch his chest. You score when you move his hand back to touch his chest without moving your feet, or when you cause him to move his feet.

Here are a few more Hawaiian games of skill, adapted for use in the backyard or local park.

Ihe Pahe'e
(Spear Sliding)

Instead of spears, use broom handles. The object is to slide them on the grass so they glide between two stakes. Set the stakes about 6 inches apart. Place the starting line back about 30 feet. Holding the broom handle at the center so its weight is balanced horizontally close to the ground, take a few steps to the starting line, as you would in bowling, and swing the "spear" at the stakes so that it slides rapidly forward. Each passage through the stakes counts for a point. You can make the game harder or easier by adjusting the distance between the stakes and/or the distance between the stakes and the starting line.

'Ulu Maika

This is similar to spear sliding except that you roll stone discs. So you need to find at least one stone that is nearly spherical in shape. A flattened sphere is ideal. Two sets of stakes, 30 feet apart, are needed. Opponents face each other at each set of stakes. The first to roll holds the stone firmly and rolls it toward the opposite set of stakes. If there is more than one stone (the Hawaiians usually use four), all are rolled and then rolled back by the opponent. Each passage through the stakes counts for a point.

Lawn Bowling

This has similarities to bowling stones as enjoyed by the ancient Hawaiians but is derived today from the British version. There are special balls used that are not quite spherical. They might be available at your sporting goods store. If not, use bowling balls or croquet balls. One ball is placed about 50 feet away as the target. You each take turns rolling your ball so that it comes to rest as close to the target ball as possible. The closest ball counts for a point.

THE KEY TO LONGER LIFE IN HAWAI'I

We have covered the main ingredients of healthful living in Hawai'i—the healthful foods, the natural medicines, the fresh air and exercise, and the *aloha* spirit.

No one of these can be singled out as the sole reason or main ingredient of Hawaiian health. The natural herbs are good. The fresh fruits, nuts and vegetables are a must. The outdoor life is invigorating and "youthifying." The *aloha* spirit is stress-dissolving.

We have one more essential ingredient to discuss.

Honolulu is a busy metropolis. Even without counting a single one of the millions of tourists who visit each year, Honolulu is at this writing the 13th largest city in the United States. The office buildings are the same as in New York, Memphis, Denver or San Francisco. So is the traffic. The diversity of business, commerce and professional services makes Honolulu just like any other cosmopolitan city.

TIME AS A HEALTH FACTOR. Yet there is one difference: Hawaiian time.

No, we do not mean that it's five hours earlier than Eastern Standard Time, four hours earlier than Central Standard Time, three hours earlier than Mountain Standard Time, and two hours earlier than Pacific Standard Time.

Hawaiian time is a life style. Schedules are made and adhered to. Appointments are made and kept. In a way. The Hawaiian way.

You can get things done tomorrow even though the schedule calls for them today. You are still on time. Hawaiian time.

You can be a half-hour late for an appointment. Don't worry. No questions asked. You are still on time. Hawaiian time.

This acceptance of elasticity rather than rigidity with regard to time is the secret ingredient of the Hawaiian life style that promotes longevity.

If you fight time all day, every day, you will have less time to fight.

If you have the time of your life all day, every day, you will have more time in your life.

The "rat race" has not come to Hawai'i . . . yet. It remains an unwanted "foreign" commodity. Hawaiians prefer Hawaiian time.

"The plane leaves in 15 minutes."

"No matter."

No matter. No rush. No tension. No sickness.

It's been fun being with you. Live naturally. Have fun. And we'll see you later. Hawaiian time.

Index

266